P9-ELD-514

IS YOUR JOB MAKING YOU FAT?

HOW TO LOSE THE OFFICE 15 ... AND MORE!

KEN LLOYD, PHD
STACEY LAURA LLOYD

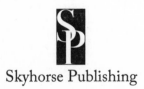

Skyhorse Publishing

CALGARY PUBLIC LIBRARY

MAR   2016

Copyright © 2016 by Ken Lloyd, PhD and Stacey Laura Lloyd

All rights reserved. No part of this book may be reproduced in any manner without the express written consent of the publisher, except in the case of brief excerpts in critical reviews or articles. All inquiries should be addressed to Skyhorse Publishing, 307 West 36th Street, 11th Floor, New York, NY 10018.

Skyhorse Publishing books may be purchased in bulk at special discounts for sales promotion, corporate gifts, fund-raising, or educational purposes. Special editions can also be created to specifications. For details, contact the Special Sales Department, Skyhorse Publishing, 307 West 36th Street, 11th Floor, New York, NY 10018 or info@skyhorsepublishing.com.

Skyhorse® and Skyhorse Publishing® are registered trademarks of Skyhorse Publishing, Inc.®, a Delaware corporation.

Visit our website at www.skyhorsepublishing.com.

10 9 8 7 6 5 4 3 2 1

Library of Congress Cataloging-in-Publication Data is available on file.

Cover design by Rain Saukas

ISBN: 978-1-63450-564-2
Ebook ISBN: 978-1-5107-0152-6

Printed in the United States of America

This book is intended as a reference volume for informational purposes only. Before engaging in any weight management or exercise program, consult first with your physician. The book's content is structured to assist you in making effective decisions about weight loss and conditioning, and it is not intended as an alternative to any advice or treatment provided by your physician. The authors and the publisher specifically disclaim any responsibility for unfavorable outcomes that may follow or result from the information provided in this book.

To Roberta Lloyd—a.k.a. Ken's wife and Stacey's mom

Contents

CHAPTER 4

Becoming Round by Sitting Around

CHAPTER 8

Traveling without Unraveling   **163**

CHAPTER 9

Conventional Strategies for Unconventional Jobs 182

CHAPTER 10
Let's Do Dinner   **209**

Introduction

When you step on your bathroom scale and take a look at the numbers, are you in disbelief? Up and up the digits fly, settling at a figure that just can't be right. But it's your figure. Your mind races. Maybe you're not standing on the right spot, so you move back an inch. No difference. Maybe the scale's broken. Fat chance. Maybe there's extra weight from your clothes. But you're in your underwear. Maybe it's time to stop saying maybe and look at the real reason why you're gaining weight. Is your job making you fat? Yes!

This weighty conclusion is not based on conjecture, anecdotes, hypotheses, or suppositions. It's based on fact. You might be wondering how this can be? If the definition of work includes labor, toil, and exertion to achieve a particular outcome, how in the world can working be fattening? It seems counterintuitive. The traditional mindset is that if you're busy working, you're burning calories. And if you're burning calories, you're going to lose weight. Unfortunately, this classical thinking has become outdated.

There have been major changes in the nature of work and the goings-on in the workplace that have turned many of today's jobs into ideal positions for putting on pounds. This largely unrecognized fact has become the elephant in the room—and if you don't take action now, that's what you'll become, too. How do you connect the dots and clearly see that your job is the cause of your burgeoning waistline? And more importantly, how do you take action to stop this ballooning trend before you pop out any further? The answers are in this book.

Take a look at today's workplaces versus those of the 1960s. Back then, places of work were a flurry of activity. Employees were up and about, carrying files from office to office, rushing from one meeting to another, and shifting paperwork and reports from here to there. Workplaces of the Sixties were a whirlwind of bustle, motion, and movement. In that era, it took a considerable amount of physical activity and energy to get most jobs done, whether they were white collar or blue.

Throughout the subsequent decades, however, the amount of physical activity associated with the vast majority of jobs has been in a steady state of decline. While approximately 50 percent of all jobs in 1960 required at least moderate physical activity, that number has dropped to a mere 20 percent today. And to make matters worse, a related finding shows that the remaining 80 percent of jobs typically call for minimal physical activity. As was spelled out in the scientific journal *PLoS One*, this transition in the workplace over the years has led to a situation where employees are burning 120 to 140 fewer calories per day when at work. And when you consider that this is happening across the United States labor force of more than 144 million workers, you start to get a much clearer idea of what's behind today's obesity epidemic—and what's behind the large behinds. After all, recent figures—so to speak—show that approximately 75 percent of men and 66 percent of women in the United States are overweight or obese.

If you picture today's workplaces, what typically comes to mind is a proliferation of cubicles with inert humans using keyboards. Fingers are getting exercise, but people aren't. Moving files and papers? It only takes a click. As for meetings? Go online or use video conferencing. Want to discuss something with your boss? Send her an email. Need to pick up the phone? Talk into your headset. Millions of jobs that used to call on employees to zip around now call for them to sit around. As a result, millions of calories are now being "waisted."

Do you sit for most of the day in front of your computer, on phone calls, and in meetings? Is your work area so ergonomically correct that you hardly need to move in order to access every conceivable item you may ever need to get your job done? If so, you're working in a perfect incubator for increasing your weight. At the same time, while being sedentary contributes to weight gain, there are many other inflationary elements that come uniquely together in the workplace and exponentially increase the likelihood that you're going to expand. The first step is to identify these causes, and the second step is to control them. Some are overt and in your face—and will ultimately lead you to stuff your face—while others are more sneaky and sinister. In combination, they team up to make you fatten up.

These figure-filling factors are spelled out in detail in the chapters that follow. While it's important to recognize the factors on your job that are making you fat, it's even more imperative to develop plans, strategies, priorities, benchmark dates, and measurement methods to successfully deal with them. There are actions you can take to lose weight right now. And keep it off for good. This isn't a diet. This isn't a fad. This is simply a matter of applying the same planning, energy, drive, focus, attention, and commitment that you place on every goal at work to the goal of preventing your job from making you fat.

The proof is in the pudding, so to speak. As was found in a landmark 2012 study conducted by CareerBuilder, after surveying more than 5,700 workers from a variety of industries, the irrefutable conclusion was that when people are at work, they tend to gain weight. In fact, of the wide range of individuals surveyed, 44 percent responded that they gained weight in their current job. The researchers also found that 26 percent of the surveyed workers gained more than ten pounds, and 14 percent gained over twenty pounds. There's even a common expression that describes the weight gain that's associated with work—it's called "the office fifteen." Much like "the freshman fifteen" referring to the typical weight gain of a college freshman adjusting to a new life of pizza and partying, the office fifteen stands for the fifteen pounds that employees are likely to gain in the first few months of taking on an office job. And worse, the odds are that they will gain even more weight over the years to come.

The obesity pandemic is not just confined to the United States, nor is the relationship between work and weight gain. There are approximately 2.1 billion overweight adults in the world, and international studies have come up with similar findings regarding working and waistlines. A two-year study of over 9,000 Australian women found that those who worked over thirty-five hours per week were more likely to gain weight than those who worked fewer hours or were outside of the workforce altogether. The message is loud and clear—the more you work, the more you gain.

The added weight that comes from your job is a lose-lose proposition for you and your employer. With the extra pounds that your job is foisting on you, there's an increased risk of cardiovascular disease, cancer, depression, type 2 diabetes, and even death. Yes, it's that serious. When you're carrying around excess weight, it can be more difficult for you to carry out your job responsibilities at peak levels. In today's competitive workplaces, any such slippage is likely to be noticed, and not in a favorable light. From the standpoint of lose-lose, you just might lose your job.

Employers also lose because of workers' weight gain—obese employees tend to be sick more often. And when people are out because of illness, there can be numerous operational problems in terms of coordination, communication, productivity, and overall output. At the same time, there can be morale issues among the other employees who have to do extra work because of the absences of coworkers. And further, there can be additional costs in insurance premiums for the employer as a result of the frequency and magnitude of medical claims.

In 2013, the American Medical Association officially declared obesity to be a disease. What's a major cause of this epidemic? Your job. Consider this book your inoculation. The only thing that should be fat on your job is your paycheck.

Chapter 1

The Corporate Foodscape

If you look around most workplaces today, you're likely to find a vast array of food that's strategically spread out from one end of a company to the other, all tempting the taste buds of unsuspecting staffers who can't help but grab a bit of this, a bite of that, a handful of those, and a plate of something else. Foods of every heart-stopping variety line the hallways, break rooms, coffee stations, coffee tables, end tables, and desks, enticing each passerby with tantalizing morsels of fat and calories. And there's no need for a special event, milestone, or accomplishment for the food to flow across organizations. The food just appears all over the place, in portions ranging from small to large. Employees readily indulge, only to find that they too have morphed from small to large.

Interestingly, one of the more common terms used across many different organizations is "cube farm," an expression that quaintly describes the acres of cubicles that now populate many corporate landscapes. While use of the word "cube" is indeed an accurate depiction of the shape of each inhabitant's habitat, the idea of a "farm" is even more telling. The reason why today's workplaces are veritable farms is that employees are constantly pigging out on more varieties of crops and crap than one could ever imagine.

THE HANDY CANDY BOWL

While employees may or may not know much about locating some fairly important destinations in their workplace, such as the lost-and-found, the nearest exit, the defibrillator, or the fire extinguishers, they all know the precise locations of every bowl of candy. Once you're in their vicinity, they're impossible to miss. The bowls are brimming with colorful delights, striking a stark and eye-catching contrast with the mundane items surrounding them. And once these caloric containers have set their roots into the workplace, it doesn't take long for them to multiply like sugar-flavored rabbits and spread across the entire company.

Locations Galore

You walk up to the front desk, and there's a candy bowl. You stop by the coffee station, and there's another. You step into your manager's office, and there's one on her desk. And while walking around may be good for you, the junk you ingest will quickly render all of those footsteps useless. The candy contents of these bowls stick to a common theme, as well as to your fingers and later to your thighs. The treats may be mini-sized, but they'll make you anything but.

The evolution of the candy bowl in most organizations starts out innocently enough. Typically, an HR staffer or manager thinks it would be sweet to have a candy bowl in the reception area, perhaps as a way to send an inviting message to visitors. For those employees who prefer to grab a handful of candy instead of dropping eighty-five cents in the vending machine down the hall, this kind of dispensary is a nice little perk. Speaking of perks, many employees will readily devour these sugary offerings because of a deep-seated belief that such consumption will perk them up and keep them energized throughout the day. Instead of dispensing candy, it's time to dispense with that myth right now. Yes, sugar can give you a brief rush of energy. However, this is soon followed by what nutritionists refer to as a "sugar crash," as sleepiness along with markedly delayed reflexes and reactions set in. Sugar's burst of energy is a bust.

Is there a candy bowl at the front desk in your company? How about at your workstation? Many managers place a bowl on their desk in order to send a message of friendliness, collaboration, and accessibility to the employees who enter their lair. For some managers, the hope is that the candy bowl will increase employee visits, while also encouraging these employees to like the managers themselves. However, if you're a manager and this is part of your strategy to build positive attitudes toward you, here's a cheery thought—research has found that managers who place an emphasis on being liked actually tend to be viewed as weak, marginally competent, dependent, and insecure. Employees would rather have managers who know their stuff, rather than managers who stuff their employees. Treating employees with respect and trust will go a lot further than treating them with treats.

It's not surprising that candy bowls that are strategically located throughout an organization have also become today's water coolers. They're magnetic congregating venues where employees stop by to chitchat and literally chew the fat. One key problem is that it's extremely difficult for even the most determined, disciplined, and diet-devoted employee to refrain from partaking when chatting with chomping coworkers at this modern day cracker barrel. After all, if you just stand there and watch your peers munch and crunch, you're likely to feel out of place, sense discomfort, and even submit yourself to some less-than-saccharine ridicule.

Succumbing to Sugar

What happens if you decide to take one little, tiny taste? You'll probably end up taking one more. And then another ... and another ... and another. How many times has this happened to you? The candy is practically addicting. It affects the pleasure pathways in your brain, and it's difficult to stop eating it once you start. In fact, many researchers contend that sugar is an addictive drug just like tobacco and alcohol. That's no sweet deal.

PUTTING THE KIBOSH ON THE CANDY BOWL

Before the candy bowl puts the bite on you, or vice versa, the key foundational concept is to approach this situation and the entire issue of weight gain on the job by establishing weight loss goals. The idea is to apply the same business mindset and skills that you use in goal-setting for any other major project at work. And this means setting real goals—not fools' goals. While it may sound convincing to say that your goal is to lose weight or even indicate that you want to lose a specific number of pounds, such statements are not goals. Rather, they're wishes and dreams. While it's nice to have them, they're not going to get you where you want to be. For goals to be effective, they need to be clear, specific, measurable, realistic, and backed up with an action plan that spells out how you're going to achieve them. This plan should include monitoring your performance along the way, benchmark dates and deadlines, strategies for making course corrections as needed, steps for accessing needed resources, and techniques for measuring how you've done. When you set objectives in the weight-loss arena—arguably the most important arena in your life—it's serious business that calls for goal-setting strategies suitable for your most serious business projects.

In supporting your efforts to get to your goal, there are several steps you can take in dealing with the candy bowl to put the lid on this matter. In the first place, the bowls don't need to be terminated—it's just their candy contents that need to be fired. One strategy is to speak with whoever replenishes these canisters and suggest a change to more figure-friendly offerings. This means taking out the sugary and fatty trash and putting in snacks that are appealing to your palate, but far less appalling to your waistline, cholesterol count, blood sugar, and caloric intake. Such offerings include low-calorie packs of dried fruits and nuts as well as low-calorie bars. All it takes to introduce them into your organization is a quick online search followed by a short email to the person filling the bowls in your company. But if you encounter resistance from your candy-committed coworkers, there are also sugar-free candies that make a tasty compromise.

Finger Food

At the same time, take a closer look at the contents of the candy bowl, specifically in terms of unpackaged items. Some companies offer treats that are devoid of any wrappers at all, and there's usually a spoon or ladle for dipping in and digging out a serving. However, you obviously know that when no one is looking, some of your associates are just sticking their fingers right in the bowl and pulling out a handful of sweets, quickly tossing their quarry into their mouths, perhaps licking a finger or two, and diving in again for a second helping. In the process, the only pieces they leave behind are the families of bacteria that ride on their fingers. The next time you're tempted to pick up the ladle and take out a spoonful of those unwrapped delicacies, just remember that you're not really dealing with a candy bowl. Rather, it's a finger bowl. And if children happen to visit your workplace and want a little treat, how many are going to use the ladle? How many even know what a ladle is? When kiddies are taking goodies out of the candy bowl, it becomes more like a dish—a Petri dish.

Looks Can Be Deceiving

However, even if the contents are wrapped, and even if they appear to be on the healthier side, that doesn't mean that you should instantly ingest. Rather, your next step is to take a second and more detailed look at whatever the offerings may be and determine how they align with your weight loss objectives—especially in terms of calories, carbohydrates, sugar, and fat. That way, you can grab an item from the candy bowl if you truly want it without abandoning your goals. Just like projects on the job, you'd monitor your progress and make sure that you're gathering all of the information you need along the way. And whether it's managing your work or your weight, some of the most powerful strategies today are technology based. Consider your smartphone your new dining advisor. There are apps that help you track your food and exercise as well as give you personalized information on how many calories to take in per day to help you manage your weight. There are also apps that let you scan the bar code of items in order to see the nutritional information and rating for a specific food. Spoiler alert—sometimes after reading the ingredients and seeing the garbage that many foods contain, you may lose your appetite altogether.

Viscerally Speaking

Want another way to survive the candy bowl blues? Listen to your gut reaction. You're always able and allowed to have a piece of candy, so these foods don't have to seem so exciting and forbidden. If your grumbling stomach is leading you to the bowl of chocolates like a voracious vulture, predetermine the item or amount you'll be taking before you get there. You'll be surprised that when you slow down, pay attention to your hunger, and stick to your planned allocation, you'll have much more control and restraint in making your selection.

Interestingly from the standpoint of listening to your stomach, research has consistently proven that many great decisions in business are made on the basis of gut feel. Use your viscera to enhance your judgment and not your waistline.

Search Party

Since the candy bowls often morph into social centers that include ingesting whatever the offerings may be, another approach is to find other venues in your organization that are free of edibles but can serve as meeting places. If you get together with colleagues in an area that's void of food, the odds of seeking out a snack diminish significantly. From the standpoint of thinking outside of the box—of candy—such a meeting place could be the parking lot or hallways where you and your associates can take a brief walk while catching up on the latest news. Instead of consuming calories, you'll be burning them. Instead of engorging your body, you'll be toning it. Instead of chewing junk, you'll be eschewing it.

Committing Yourself

There are further preemptive steps that you can take to prevent the ballooning problems that emanate from the infamous bowl. One way to help yourself refrain from engaging in a candy bowl binge is to write a contract with yourself. Research has found that this is one of the easiest and most effective ways to introduce a behavioral change, break a habit, and improve performance on the job. Similarly, these contracts can be equally efficacious in helping you control your weight. And they can be even more powerful if you write them out by hand. A contract can be as basic as, "I won't eat any more of the free candy that's provided. If I want candy, I'm going to buy it." Doing some actual writing engages different muscles and brain activity when compared with punching out a few words on your keyboard. As a result, these actions have an increased likelihood of sticking with you and impacting your future behavior.

Also, by committing to buy such foods with your own money rather than consuming them because they're free, you're engaging in two additional strategies that help curtail this self-destructive behavior. First, there's some pain associated with spending money when you know you can obtain the offerings at no cost. By committing to only acquire candy by expending your personal funds, you're associating the painful activity of spending your own money with the acquisition of the candy, and that can help you refrain from making the purchase. On a more subtle level, eating this type of junk is literally and figuratively going to cost you. That little message can also help introduce more restraint into your thinking. Instead of a candy bowl on your desk, keep a money bowl and deposit your unused vending machine change in there. By the end of the month or months, you can see how much you saved not only in cash, but in calories as well. Plus, you can take this money and use it to buy something that helps your body instead of harms it—such as an article of clothing in a smaller size.

And speaking of contracts, there are even websites that enable you to take this concept to the next level by engaging your friends and relatives to support you. On some of these websites, you can establish work-related contracts that focus on streamlining various aspects of your job, meeting a particular sales goal, or gaining an additional certification in your area of expertise. Similarly, you can make weight-related contracts that focus on exercising daily, refraining from eating out of the candy bowl, or obtaining specific weight-loss results.

Candy Toss

If you're thinking about having a candy bowl on your desk, regardless of its contents, here's an idea. Don't! If it's on your desk, it's within arm's reach—and guess who's going to be doing most of the eating? Plus, if you're working while sticking your hand into a bowl of food throughout the day, it's almost impossible to keep track of how much you're actually eating. You don't need food of any kind to be constantly staring at you in the face, daring you to resist the seductively sweet or savory goodness that's just one bite away. Besides, if this tub of temptation weren't on your desk, you wouldn't necessarily be having this mental joust in the first place. By keeping these containers of candy at a distance, the desire to indulge will drop—and your weight is more likely to follow suit.

COUNTERS FILLED WITH CRAP

In addition to the countless candy bowls strewn from one corner table of an organization to the other, there are also baked, boiled, broiled, steamed, stewed, and deep-fried concoctions engaged in heated or unheated competition with them. As in the case of candy bowls, these offerings celebrate nothing. Not a birthday. Not an achievement. Not a landmark. Not a special event. Rather, they simply appear. And then they simply disappear, but not from your waistline.

Bagel Basics

One of the most popular items put out for employees is the platter of bagels. A bagel may look harmless, but don't be fooled. The fact that bagels are shaped like zeros says it all, and yet their calories and carb count are anything but zero. A bagel is essentially four pieces of bread—bread that's low in vitamins, minerals, and fiber. It typically contains at least fifty grams of carbohydrates, and as soon as they hit your system, they quickly morph into their evil twin—sugar. And here's the topper. When employees select a topping for their bagel, they usually smear even more fat and calories by adding cream cheese or butter. Then, as if this concoction isn't sufficiently damaging to the waistline, the final ingredient, jelly, gets slopped on top—adding at least fifty more calories and ten more grams of carbohydrates, and that's if you only add a tablespoon. But, be serious. Can you even measure a tablespoon-sized serving of this sugar-gel with a knife? So you simply slop on an amount that looks right to you. But take a real good look at the round and doughy shape of a bagel. The more you consume, the more bagel-like you'll become. You are what you eat.

Donut Duty

Another frequent occupant of the platter of fatter matter is the ubiquitous donut. Once again, here's a treat that's usually shaped like a zero, clearly symbolizing its nutritional value. However, a donut should really be shaped like a minus sign since it undermines your health in so many different ways—actually, the long donuts come close to representing this. In the first place, donuts typically contain the troika of ingredients that are destructive to the human body—sugar, white flour, and trans fat. What's the problem with trans fats? Not much if your goal is to increase your LDL cholesterol (the bad type), decrease your HDL (the good type), and increase your chances of coronary heart disease. By the way, one donut's calorie count can easily hit 400 or more. If you still feel like digging into one of those warm, mouthwatering, and perfectly textured donuts perched so delicately on the platter just outside of your cube, here's one more little tidbit to keep in mind—donuts are prepared at very high temperatures, and evidence suggests that consuming foods that have been made this way may increase a person's risk of developing various cancers.

If your reasoning for devouring these sweet treats is because you work hard, and heck, you deserve them, it's time to take a couple of steps back and get some perspective. A self-chosen reward shouldn't be a self-inflicted surge of bodily harm and guilt. Apply a little logic and foresight. Are you going to feel rewarded a few minutes or even seconds after you lick that last morsel of powdered sugar from your fingers? Get real. You're going to feel like crap because you ate crap. The next time you come face-to-face with a donut, just think of what you're looking at. Donut. Just change the "u" to an "o." When you see a donut, think "do not."

Tricky Treats

This same type of thinking applies to the other sugar bombs that are dropped on plates, platters, and dishes throughout so many organizations today. Some of these indelicacies include coffee cakes, sweet rolls, and cinnamon buns, all dished out to the employees simply for the sake of doing so. The idea is that if there's even a hint of room on a table, counter, desktop, or shelf, it would be a corporate sin to let it just sit there when it could be adorned with sinful sweets.

There's a certain irony in the actual names of some of these goodies. Coffee cake doesn't contain any of the antioxidants or disease-fighting power that's found in real coffee. A sweet roll is actually a roll of fat, and once it lands in your stomach, it's going to stay there. Not such a sweet outcome, is it? And you shouldn't be fooled by the specious façade posited by the cinnamon bun. Nutritionists regard cinnamon as one of the healthiest and most beneficial spices in the world. But by partnering with the bun, everything but the cinnamon is fattening, unhealthy, or both. So when you're weighing the pros and cons about eating one or two or more, think less about the cinnamon and more about the buns—namely your own.

COUNTERING THE OFFERINGS ON THE COUNTER

Fortunately, there are all sorts of steps that you can take in order to avoid the pound-producing pottage that's piled up on so many corporate counters. Speaking literally, the best steps when faced with these weighty matters are those that take you in another direction. After all, for you to partake in bagels, donuts, cinnamon buns, and the like, you need to amble over to the counter where they're perched. Thus, one solution is for you to refrain from walking anywhere near them—simply use an alternate route or walk on by and don't make eye contact with the food. If you stop to just take a look, the assault on your senses can be too much to resist. Don't sabotage yourself! You wouldn't undercut the progress you've made in pursuing your work goals, so why do so when pursuing your weight goals?

Exploring Options

At the same time, when resolving issues or concerns at work, it's best to focus on problems rather than symptoms. Instead of taking detours and dealing with the symptoms of this situation, another option is to deal with the cause—the unhealthy food-stuff. After all, there are far healthier alternatives to the scale-tipping tripe that's proffered up in so many workplaces today. If your company is intent on giving out bagels, there are healthier options within the realm of bagel-hood. Many bagel chains and shops are now offering tasty low-fat, whole grain, and whole wheat options, all with significantly lower calorie counts. Also, there are store-bought bagels that can be far healthier than the standard fare. Plus, instead of smothering these bagels or any others with high-fat and high-calorie toppings, how about going with nonfat cream cheese, trans-fat-free buttery spreads, and low-calorie jellies, jams, and preserves? Simple swap-outs go a long way. And further, try using an actual measuring utensil such as a real tablespoon, rather than simply using a generic plastic knife, spoon, or shovel to smother your bagel with toppings. As another strategy, why not add some hummus, tomatoes, onions, cucumbers, and avocado to your bagel?

Splitting Time

Another strategy to cut calories and fat in these sweet treats is to do some actual cutting—that is, split them into halves, thirds, or fourths. You can always enjoy these items if you truly want them, but try eating a smaller portion. Dig out the softer insides of a bagel and just eat the firmer crust. Cut out the center of the piece of coffee cake and just eat the exterior. And speaking of downsizing, how about suggesting that your company provides smaller portions in the first place, such as small or thin bagels, donut holes, or mini cinnamon buns? Smaller portions won't automatically induce employees to take more of the items, since doing so can easily send out a message of unmitigated gluttony. Even if some of your coworkers regard the smaller portions as an invitation to double-up or even triple-up, there's no law that forces you to do so. Besides, if you really want to get smaller, smaller portions are a great way to go.

To Your Health

Without too much hunting, you can also find healthier donuts, cinnamon buns, and coffee cakes. No, that's not an oxymoron. Vegan varieties are sold across the country, and as you probably guessed, there are apps—for your appetite—that can help you locate vegetarian and vegan vendors near you. Additionally, by exploring your local supermarket or by searching online for specialty donut and sweet shops, you can locate all sorts of goodies that are low-calorie, sugar-free, fat-free, and gluten-free, as well as made with mashed banana, unsweetened applesauce, and honey rather than outrageous amounts of butter and sugar—all that's missing are the calories and remorse. You don't have to make sacrifices, just make substitutions. What you're left with are healthier and arguably tastier goodies than the run-of-the-mill desserts that bombard you at work. Now is the time to meet with whoever's making the culinary choices in your organization and suggest some healthier alternatives. And if you're the person who actually makes the selections, why wait any longer to change company practices?

Of course, there's a more fundamental question that needs to be addressed as well. If your company is going to put out scads of food across the organizational horizon, why not start out with food that's inherently better for employees in the first place, rather than having to resort to sugar-free this and low-calorie that? Instead of the baked or deep-fried artery-cloggers, how about fruit, nuts, yogurt, and other popular and healthy choices? After all, it's a little nutty for an organization to ignore healthy options.

CALORIES FROM COWORKERS

Another weighty source of fattening foods is your fellow employees. In celebration or commemoration of nothing whatsoever, gaggles of coworkers take delight in bringing all sorts of food-stuffs to the workplace and sharing them with anyone who's inclined to partake. These edible goodies or "baddies" are found lining the hallways, taking a prominent position on the donors' desks, and spread across the break room.

Since such edible offerings aren't associated with any particular event or landmark, one immediate question is why various employees are inclined to bring in these foods in the first place. Some employees bear such gifts because they want to be well liked. While it's obviously better to be liked than disliked, there are a couple of flaws associated with connecting food distribution to personal likability. First, there's no reason to assume that bestowing treats on fellow employees is going to generate positive feelings from them. Even if coworkers like the baked goods, that doesn't mean they'll like the baker. Secondly, the actual reasons why employees like their coworkers tend to be focused more on behavior in the workplace than in the supermarket or kitchen. Truly positive feelings toward coworkers are far more heavily based on such factors as competence, cooperation, reliability, and honesty.

Just Being Friendly

For other employees, the primary reason for bringing in food for you and your coworkers is simply to do something nice. Of course, as well intentioned as this gesture may be, the reality is that such victuals can be rather vicious in terms of their impact on your body, especially since these offerings tend to be long on waistline-enhancers. Although the baker is bestowing these homegrown creations out of the goodness of her heart, they're soon to result in the badness of yours.

In Pursuit of Praise

Then there are the cadres of cooks who bring in food right from their own kitchens, motivated by less benign factors. One is to demonstrate some superiority over you and your associates. Perhaps this employee's job performance isn't particularly stellar, and a demonstration of culinary competence is a way to jump up a few notches in everyone's eyes. A related need that homemade dishes satisfy for your cooking colleagues is that their offerings generate an opportunity for attention, recognition, and accolades. For many such employees, this is an easy way to receive "oohs" and "ahhhs" at work.

Think Twice

If you're thinking about ingesting some of these home-brewed or stewed concoctions, keep in mind that you have very little information about the ingredients. Who knows how much sugar, butter, and salt are in that fried catfish or sweet-and-sour pork? And if you ask, you're likely to receive generalities, often in terms of a pinch of this, a dash of that, and a dollop of something else. The outcome may taste good, but it's likely to do you no good whatsoever. As a side note, you also have no information regarding the cleanliness practices of your coworker chef and the sanitation levels in the kitchen from which this creation emerged. Who knows how long the chicken cacciatore was perched on the counter at your colleague's home? How long did it sit in the car, bus, or train on its way to work? How long has it been parked in the break room for viewing?

Lovely Leftovers

There's also a category of food that's intended for the home audience but still makes its way to the workplace. Somehow, there are employees who think that last night's—or last week's—leftover meatloaf that resembles a roadkill is just what their coworkers want. Leftovers suffer from all of the potential problems associated with the home-baked concoctions, except for one important point. Leftovers are just that . . . left over. Who knows when they were made, how they were made, who had their hands in them, and why they weren't consumed in the first place? Employees who bring leftovers to work typically ask themselves, "Should I bring what's left of this corned beef hash to work, or should I just throw it out?" It all boils down to the break room or the trash bin.

Do you really want to eat anything that came perilously close to landing in a dumpster?

Repeat Performances

There are times when offerings from home are items that were originally given to your coworkers, rather than prepared by them. These are the classic re-gifts that go unopened from house to house, only to end up one day in your workplace. And by the way, sometimes these items hibernate for extended periods in your coworker's pantry, only to show up on the job far after their expiration date. If you're interested in extending your own expiration date, these mysterious morsels should be avoided.

Kids in the Kitchen

Another offering that makes its way from the home to the workplace is the creation that's made by your coworker and his kids. By definition, these concoctions are not likely to be healthy. After all, how many parents go to the kitchen for a fun activity with their children and reach for the broccoli, cabbage, or kale? Rather, a project in the kitchen with kids usually means a hyperglycemic amalgam of sugar, frosting, sprinkles, and chocolate chips, all glued together with white flour and butter into heart-stopping nuggets for you and your coworkers to devour. While these baked goods may look and smell delicious, they're typically fattening, artery clogging, blood sugar boosting, and blood pressure raising. But if you feel yourself buckling to the temptation—and forget about buckling your pants—here's another point to keep in mind. Have you ever seen kids in the kitchen during these projects? There's plenty of finger licking, spoon licking, and bowl licking, and sometimes these parent-child cooking activities take place when the child is sick and home from school. After all, this type of activity cheers up the child. So there's a little sneezing, coughing, and nose blowing all over the food. If you're thinking about eating these homemade delights, you might want to think about getting a flu shot first.

THE PEER PRESSURE COOKER

On a broader basis, the issue of peer pressure is a real problem when you're trying to avoid weight gain on the job. When you don't indulge in the food that's being given out, you can be subjected not only to sneers but also to a barrage of derogatory comments and innuendoes, along with unending cajoling and imploring for you to join the engorging. Since peer pressure plays such a critical role in shaping employee attitudes and behavior in myriad work-related situations, there are a couple of points to keep in mind when such pressure is applied to food consumption. If you succumb even once to this pressure to sample that homemade quiche, chocolate cake, or jambalaya, you've shown your coworkers that if they keep badgering you, you'll give in at some point. After all, by capitulating and taking a plateful of peach cobbler, you're rewarding the behavior of your pressure-playing peers. In addition, since people tend to repeat behaviors that are rewarded, you can expect similar pressure from them down the road. This means that you need to show real restraint in the face of relentless peer pressure to dive into the cornucopia. If you continuously refrain from bending to their pressure, they're ultimately going to stop trying to push you and your palate.

What if your persistent peers simply thrust a plate of pottage into your hands? Obviously, it would be rude to push it back or make a scene. In this situation, your best strategy is to simply take whatever's being offered, while recognizing that there's no rule that you have to eat it. And as you probably remember from your childhood days, there's an art to moving food around a plate so that it looks like you have been nibbling away. No matter who's pushing you to eat this or that, you're the boss when it comes to the food you consume. If you're going to partake, the decision has to be made by you, not your peers.

Ulterior Motives

An additional factor behind your coworkers' desire to inundate the workplace with foodstuffs for your personal engorgement doesn't stem from altruism, personal generosity, or a need for recognition, but rather from something more sinister. These are the employees who show up with enticing fat-laden assortments in order to sabotage the weight loss efforts, actions, and goals of their peers. Is it jealousy? Insecurity? Immaturity? Whatever the cause, treat these saboteurs just as you'd treat anyone who's trying to undercut your performance, productivity, or success on the job. Don't let these people get to you. Don't let these people pressure you or embarrass you. Rather, let these people inspire you to work even harder.

Extra, Extra!

Lastly, be aware of the random snack attack email or PA announcement telling you something like, "Jennifer baked cookies and brownies! Come by the break room!" What should you do when this info hits your inbox or your ears? One strategy is to ignore it. You're busy, you have work to do, so just pass. After all, if you head down to the break room, you'll be putting yourself directly in the line of temptation and subjected to peer pressure. The reality is that you don't rush to the supermarket or department store every time you receive a mailer or hear an advertisement, so why should you feel compelled to rush to the break room in response to a similar pitch at work?

At the same time, if you want to go, take a moment to process what's going on here. How hungry are you? Decide right then and there if you're going to participate. And if so, reasonably predetermine the amount that you're going to eat, and stick to that commitment. If you head to the break room and start eating before you've clearly thought about what you're going to ingest, you're very likely to open the floodgates and ingest in excess. This is simply a case of managing your hunger and managing yourself.

VISITORS AND YOUR VISCERA

It might surprise you that guests, visitors, vendors, and customers can all contribute to your weight gain at work. How? Through the gifts and offerings they bring when meeting with you or others in the company. Even if you never interact with anyone from the outside world in your job, many of your fellow employees do. And when they receive edible gifts, they may consume some, while placing others on a counter or in the break room for you and your associates to gobble up.

In addition to applying the same strategies that you'd use to prevent overindulging in the foodstuffs brought in by your fellow employees, there are a couple of additional points to consider when dealing with food from outsiders. When these goodies appear, you don't have to eat them. They usually arrive unexpectedly, and if they weren't in your work area right now, you wouldn't be thinking about stuffing your face with them. Additionally, your company probably has a policy regarding gifts from outsiders which indicates that employees are to refrain from accepting them from suppliers, vendors, and the like. It would be helpful to advise these gift-bestowing outsiders of this fact. If they persist, you should consider donating their offerings to a charitable organization in your area.

George Mallory, a famous mountaineer from the early twentieth century, was once asked why he wanted to climb Mount Everest. His reputed answer was, "Because it's there." If that's your rationale for eating the food that randomly appears at your job, you can plan on looking like Mount Everest.

Chapter 2

Don't Let the Morning Eat You for Breakfast

"Breakfast is the most important meal of the day." Sound familiar? You've probably heard the saying before. Multiple times. It's been ingrained in your mind since you were a child. And in actuality, there's definitely some truth behind it, as studies have consistently proven that eating a healthy breakfast directly benefits your general well-being, overall cognition, as well as your weight. And yet countless employees neglect to incorporate any breakfast, let alone a healthy breakfast, into their workday routine. A 2011 study revealed that thirty-one million Americans skip breakfast each day, and a survey of British office workers revealed that a third of them skip breakfast, with nearly 17 percent who never have breakfast and 17 percent who have it just one to three times per week. And for those who are able to grab a bite, all too often these morning meals tend to consist of muffin mishaps, donut disasters, and bacon binges. The irony is that whether you're a person who tends to skip breakfast or one who usually downs breakfast foods full of sugar, carbs, and fat, the result is invariably the same—both actions are linked to obesity. The concern is that as workers place precedence on their jobs over their breakfasts, the only thing they end up gaining is weight. But don't dismay, as there are numerous attack strategies to conquer the breakfast battle and win this game of scones.

THE BREAKFAST BREAKUP

Breakfast has lost its priority in the morning routine of numerous working people today, and the reasons behind this trend are piling up like hotcakes. One of the main culprits causing breakfast to get put on the back burner is simply a matter of technology. Employees today are always connected to their work, and the first thing that most of them do as soon as they wake up is head straight to their smartphone, tablet, or laptop, even before they head to the bathroom. In fact, the average American worker starts checking his email in bed at around 7:09 a.m., and by 8:00 a.m., nearly seven in ten workers have gone through their email. In a word, where there's WiFi, there's work. So you're busy consuming information instead of consuming a healthy morning meal. Technology also plays a role in determining when many of today's jobs actually start, since the globalization of the corporate world has made it so that no matter where you are, you need to be on the same schedule as others in different time zones. If you're checking overseas markets, communicating with colleagues across the country, or even working in an industry that caters to customers who are up at the crack of dawn, you're unlikely to find yourself cracking an egg for a sunny-side up breakfast before the sun is even out. Many jobs today, from hospital staffers to coffee shop baristas, have incredibly early call times that may be hard to stomach, so workers end up putting nothing in their stomachs at all.

Time Troubles

Another breakfast buzzkill is simply the matter of not having enough time. Employees feel that they're so strapped in the morning that they can't possibly take care of all of their responsibilities as well as incorporate a healthy meal before heading off to work. Packing your daughter's lunch. Finding your son's soccer cleats. Letting the dog out. Deciding what to wear. Blow-drying your hair. Putting away the dishes. Taking out the trash. Letting the dog in. What's the weather again? The morning is a hectic blur because of a seemingly endless list of pre-work responsibilities. So it's somehow acceptable to either forgo feeding yourself at all or rely on quick-toasting or microwaveable calorific crap to appease you and the members of your household. And of course, there's the all-too-tempting snooze button, which can get more hits than a punching bag. Plenty of workers devote their precious morning minutes to clinging to those final fleeting moments of sleep. But all too often, these last seconds spent enjoying a warm bed can mean that you won't have time to enjoy a warm bowl of oatmeal later. If this is a trade-off that you're making each workday, it can be said that when you snooze, you lose everything but weight.

BREAKFAST BACKFIRES

The reality is that as working people consistently fail to recognize the importance of eating a healthy breakfast, they're consistently putting themselves at risk for weight gain as well as a host of other health concerns. As many studies have shown, skipping breakfast is associated with obesity, yet there's a myth perpetuated by desperate dieters who believe that skipping breakfast is an effective way to cut calories and lose weight. But it's pretty much a weight loss bust instead of a weight loss must. All too often, your increased hunger will take over later in the workday, and you'll find yourself hovering around the vending machine like a voracious vulture. When looking at the word "breakfast" itself, you can see more of its real meaning, as it's literally a "breaking of the fast" that humans take as they sleep. But by neglecting to eat breakfast and therefore prolonging this fast for hours after you get up, you're straining your body in a way that can cause blood pressure issues, higher cholesterol levels, and an increased resistance to insulin. Not surprisingly, skipping breakfast can increase your risk of developing type 2 diabetes, as shown in a study published in the *American Journal of Clinical Nutrition*. Getting down to the heart of the matter, a study from Harvard School of Public Health revealed that men who repeatedly skipped breakfast had a 27 percent higher chance of a heart attack or death from coronary heart disease than men who ate breakfast regularly. Skipping breakfast as a dieting tactic can leave you with nothing more than dead weight.

Breakfast and Your Brain

Another non-breakfast snag has to do with your mental state. Studies have shown that people who regularly consume breakfast tend to have lower rates of depression, lower emotional malaise, and lower perceived stress levels. Plus, cognitive functions such as mental sharpness, problem-solving abilities, concentration levels, and creative thinking are all negatively impacted when you negate to have breakfast, and the same for your overall energy and coordination. A study at the University of Bath found that people who eat breakfast have a higher energy expenditure in daily physical activity over a six-week time frame when compared with those who waited to eat until noon, further demonstrating that eating breakfast supports a worker's lifestyle and supports your desire to perform at the highest level. It's also been shown that people scored 15 percent lower on memory tests when they didn't eat breakfast. Try to remember that. And here's the kicker, according to data from the Office for National Statistics and the Center for Economics and Business Research, it's been estimated that employees who skip breakfast are actually costing companies around $12.6 billion as well as 46.5 million lost working days due to the lower productivity, inferior mental focus, and poorer health and mood.

Morning Sugar

If you're the type of individual who consistently eats breakfast, but your breakfasts consistently consist of caloric concoctions full of sugar, carbs, and fat, your pre-work meal is working against you big-time. By filling your mornings with donuts, bagels, bear claws, and cinnamon rolls, you're setting the stage—and table— for an increased risk of heart disease, liver problems, type 2 diabetes, and of course, obesity. Even serial cereal eaters are at risk of committing major breakfast blunders, as many cereals on the market today can be notoriously unhealthy. You can find cereals that are more than 50 percent sugar by weight, along with many others which are more appropriately suited for the dessert aisle. The plethora of problems for your body and your brain that stem from consuming too much sugar can hurt you work-wise and weight-wise. As shown by researchers at the David Geffen School of Medicine at UCLA, consuming large amounts of sugar impairs cognitive function and your ability to learn and retain information. Not the best way to take on the workday.

Fat Facts

In a similar vein, if you're hogging the bacon, sausage, and ham each morning, you're also engaging in risky breakfast business before heading off to your business. They may be fast to fire up on the stove or in the microwave, but as multiple studies have found, these fatty foods are linked to obesity. With Americans each consuming around eighteen pounds of bacon per year, this pig problem is a big problem. These foods are full of saturated fat and cholesterol, both of which can increase your risk of stroke, plus the fact that eating processed meats can also raise your likelihood of dying from cancer and heart disease. And if that doesn't take your breath away, consuming cured meats is also linked to pulmonary disease. Perhaps it was the three little pigs that were huffing and puffing instead of the wolf. Your cognitive abilities also suffer when you consume processed meats, as these foods promote the production of the toxins in the body that can cause inflammation and plaque to accumulate in the brain. It's not surprising that bacon, ham, and smoked meats have all been tied to memory loss, dementia, and Alzheimer's disease. And who could forget the study by Harvard School of Public Health which showed that processed meat consumption was also associated with a lower sperm count? Just think of that the next time you say, "Pass the sausage."

BRINGING BACK BREAKFAST

The good news is that no matter how busy you are and how large your workload, you can always include a healthy breakfast that can prevent you from becoming large. The strategic approach is to gather all of the facts about your pre-work demands, preferences, and time commitments and then establish a schedule in order to transform your morning from chaos to calm and enable you to integrate the ideal meal. This type of forethought and planning is no different from how you'd prepare for any other work assignment or task. First, look at the time that you usually get up out of bed. Are you giving yourself ample time to get your junk done, or are you a snooze button junkie? If hitting the alarm is causing you to be late to work, it's time to end this losing breakfast battle of beating the clock once and for all. Instead, set your alarm to go off earlier so you can still satisfy the desire to hit the snooze a few times, without blowing right past your wakeup time and blowing off breakfast. The reality is that consuming a healthy breakfast will give you far more energy to take on the workday than hanging onto those last minutes of pseudo-sleep. Consider this your wakeup call.

Getting Up for the Challenge

If the time you spend connected to your smartphone, tablet, or laptop each morning is the disconnect between you and a healthy breakfast, it's your responsibility to account for this online time when you build your breakfast strategy. How much of your pre-work routine is spent scrolling through emails, reviewing reports, and taking stock of stocks? Newsflash! Gobbling up the news is not an excuse to forgo gobbling up a healthy breakfast. The same goes for the morning children challenge. Preparing your kids for school is not a justification for you to just give up breakfast, especially since incorporating a healthy breakfast into the morning routines of all the members of your household has never been so important, whether they're heading to a boardroom or a classroom. Studies indicate that children and adolescents who consume breakfast are more likely to perform better on exams, have improved memory skills, and even have higher rates of school attendance than students who go without. Plus, children who eat breakfast are more inclined to make better food choices throughout the day and have a lower risk of developing high cholesterol and obesity. But it's not only about making a healthy breakfast for your children to eat, but for you to partake as well. Studies show that children mimic the eating patterns of their parents, and when you skip breakfast and/or make unhealthy food choices for yourself, you're setting your children up to do the same.

Egging You On

What's your best bet when it comes to breakfast? There are numerous options to choose from, as a healthy breakfast doesn't mean a boring breakfast. Nutritionists contend that including protein and fiber into your morning routine can help you feel fuller longer and can help satisfy your hunger until lunch. One powerful protein option at breakfast is eggs, and they can play a grade-A role in weight management. As presented in the *Journal of the American College of Nutrition*, women who ate a breakfast consisting of eggs felt more satiated throughout the day and consumed fewer calories than women who ate a bagel-based breakfast of equal caloric value and weight. Similar results were also noted in a study by researchers at the Pennington Biomedical Research Center who found that when compared to overweight women who ate a bagel breakfast of equivalent calories and volume, overweight women who ate two eggs for breakfast as part of a low-fat/lower-cal diet also lost 65 percent more weight than the bagel eaters, reduced their waist circumference, as well as reported higher levels of energy. It should also be noted that the egg-eaters in this study didn't have any significant increase in their cholesterol or triglyceride levels, as many people shy away from eating eggs because of the cholesterol in the yolk. But don't fly the coop just yet, as research is still going on in this area. One study demonstrated that egg consumption had no effect on the cholesterol levels of 115 adults, ranging in age from thirty to sixty, along with a separate study reported in the *Journal of Nutrition* which revealed that overweight men who ate eggs as part of low-carb diet actually increased their HDL levels. Isn't it time you take a crack at having eggs for breakfast? A tasty way to enjoy eggs in the morning is to make an omelet or scramble and include your favorite vegetables and even leftover white meat chicken or turkey. Plus, with liquid egg whites sold in super-markets today, you can easily cut valuable minutes out of your prep and cleanup time with a simple pour into your pan. It's a low-cal, low-maintenance, and fast-cooking breakfast for your fast-paced pre-work morning.

Cereal Fanatics

There's also good news for cereal fans, as this quick and easy morning meal can help you reach your weight goals as long as you don't get bowled over by the plethora of unhealthy choices. As noted by Harvard researchers, eating cereals for breakfast that contain at least six grams of fiber and no more than ten grams of sugar per serving can help lower a man's likelihood of developing heart disease, type 2 diabetes, colon cancer, intestinal polyps, and even a risk of stroke. Studies have also found that adults who eat cereal tend to have healthier body weights, lower BMIs (Body Mass Index), as well as improved nutrient profiles. Don't get boxed in by unhealthy boxes—look instead for selections that are high in fiber, low in sugar, and have at least five grams of protein.

It's also important to avoid the common cereal traps that can trip you up and up your weight. First, neglecting to place an emphasis on portion size is a cereal don't, so be sure to use a measuring cup when placing the suggested serving size of cereal into your bowl. All too often, the size of your bowl may be giving you a skewed view of how much cereal you're actually consuming. Secondly, keep in mind the amount of milk you're pouring into your bowl, as many people flood their cereal or continue to add more while they eat. Again, be mindful of the serving size and measure out the exact amount. It's also important to select a nonfat milk or try sampling other healthy options such as unsweetened soy milk and almond milk. Next, pay attention to the calorie count of any other items you may be adding to your cereal. If you're used to loading your bowl with dried fruit like raisins, try adding fresh berries like blueberries, raspberries, or strawberries instead since they have more water content than their dried counterparts and can actually help you feel fuller. Plus, berries contain the antioxidant anthocyanin whose high consumption has been associated with a lower risk of heart attack in young and middle-aged women. If you're a cereal nut-adder, it's also important to pay attention to portion size, as nuts can be huge calorie contributors. Just don't go nuts. Meticulousness and precision go a long way when it comes to your workload and cereal-load.

Turning Up the Heat

Don't overlook the hot options that can fill you and your morning bowl. Not only can you heat up the milk that you add to your cereal, you can go with hot cereal varieties such as oatmeal and oat bran. Heart-healthy breakfast foods made from whole oats contain a soluble fiber known as beta-glucan that helps reduce LDL cholesterol. Oats are a good source of potassium and omega-3s, and they may also lower your risk of coronary artery disease, type 2 diabetes, and colorectal cancer. Not surprisingly, oats play a crucial role in weight management. In fact, eating oatmeal has been shown to help control your appetite and increase feelings of fullness. While there are instant oatmeal brands that you can purchase—look for unsweetened options—your best bet is to buy slow-cooking steel cut oats or rolled oats. But how can you include a slow-paced breakfast into your fast-paced morning? Stop letting the demands of your job keep you from enjoying the right kind of breakfast that your body needs. While oats take approximately fifteen minutes to cook, just like in the workplace, you can multitask while they sit stovetop, or you can apply your executive planning skills and implement a strategy, such as cooking the oats in bulk over the weekend, separating them into serving size portions for the days of the week, placing them in the refrigerator, and then reheating them individually each morning. Preparing ahead of time and nailing down a pre-work system that works for you will not only make your life easier, but healthier as well.

Sweet Replacements

For all you donut-devouring, muffin-minded, bagel-bingers out there, it's time to get real. You're too smart, with too much to offer, and work too hard to be lured in by these nutrient-empty and calorie-full offerings. Come on! You're better than this. While lower-cal versions of these foodstuffs are available today, there are other healthy options that can take their place. Start by replacing these carby and fatty food failures with items such as a healthier bread, and that means getting your butt to a supermarket and actually sorting through loaves, picking up packages, and examining labels. Look for options that say 100 percent whole wheat or 100 percent whole grain, and the first ingredient listed should read "100% whole wheat flour" or simply "whole wheat flour." Whole grains make a great addition to your morning meal since they're full of fiber, vitamins, minerals, protein, and they're lower in fat and don't contain cholesterol. Plus, whole grains have been linked to reducing the risk of heart disease, type 2 diabetes, stroke, and . . . obesity! You can still satisfy your sweet tooth tendencies and/or your desire for something crunchy by topping the whole grain bread or toast with almond butter or peanut butter. Both of these spreads are great sources of protein, have monounsaturated fat (the good fat), fiber, vitamins, and minerals. They also contain compounds known as phytosterols which can block cholesterol absorption and have been shown to lower your total cholesterol up to 10 percent and your LDL cholesterol up to 14 percent. "Nut" too shabby! If you wise up regarding the serving sizes of these scrumptious spreads and select options that don't contain loads of sugar, sodium, or other ingredients that'll cost you weight-wise, you'll benefit health-wise.

A Matter of Liquidity

It's also crucial to avoid getting lost in the morning juice jungle as you'll only come out looking like a tree stump. One of the biggest breakfast trip-ups that can up the scale is the constant slurping up of fruit juices. While juices such as orange juice are great sources of vitamin C, you're also taking in more calories and sugar than you'd like to see. In fact, simply eating an orange is around half the calories of drinking a glass of orange juice, plus the actual orange provides you with bulk and fiber which can help you feel fuller longer. If you still feel the need to break out the breakfast juices, water them down if possible, as water is and will always be the drink of champions. If your pre-work drink of choice is milk, you may want to think twice before you guzzle down glass after glass after glass. Sure, it's been ingrained in your head since youth that milk is your body's BFF as it's loaded with calcium, vitamin D, and phosphorus which are good for your bones. However, a 2014 study conducted by researchers at Uppsala University in Sweden followed more than 100,000 Swedes for up to twenty-three years, and not only was it determined there was no link between drinking milk and a decreased risk of bone fractures, these researchers also found that milk drinkers were more likely to die at younger ages than those who drank little to no milk. The issue at hand is the nutrient D-galactose, as this is what your body produces when it breaks down lactose—the sugar in milk. But D-galactose causes inflammation and a lower immune response in animals, and it's actually what scientists give to animals to imitate the effects of aging. When it comes to milk, the advice is simply to be mindful of the amount you're consuming each day.

Coffee Conundrum

And then there's coffee. It seems to be the lifeblood of countless hardworking professionals, with 54 percent of Americans over the age of eighteen drinking coffee every day, and nearly 65 percent of them drinking their coffee at breakfast. Coffee is what most of the working population depends upon in order to take on the workday. Not surprisingly, a multitude of studies throughout the years continue to weigh the pros and cons of coffee consumption, and it's time you should, too, so you don't end up weighing more. As noted in the 2012 *Harvard Health Letter*, research has shown that drinking coffee in moderation—a few cups per day—can be beneficial to your health. Coffee can lower your risk of Parkinson's disease, liver disease, and cancer. And when it comes to your job, drinking coffee has also been shown to improve cognitive abilities as well as increase your energy levels. In fact, a study in the *New England Journal of Medicine* determined that coffee drinking has even been linked to a longer life. That's something to drink to!

However, the beneficial effects of drinking coffee don't go without some heated debate. Coffee drinking has been known to cause increased blood pressure, elevated heart rate, as well as irregular heartbeat, and coffee's acidity has been linked to gastroesophageal reflux disease (GERD), heartburn, and digestive issues. There are also some differing opinions regarding coffee's impact on blood sugar, as some studies point out that your likelihood of developing type 2 diabetes is lower if you're a coffee drinker while others argue that the caffeine in coffee actually lowers your sensitivity to insulin and makes it harder for your body to control blood sugar. It's also been noted that only a quarter of America's coffee drinkers take it black, as many working people put loads of sugar, cream, and all the fattening flavors, powders, syrups, and additions into their coffee and therefore put on loads of weight. People also are getting mugged by their coffee when it's the only item they're ingesting for breakfast. Time to spill the coffee beans—this is a huge mistake. The bottom line is that coffee is made up of many powerful compounds and different components whose effects are still being studied, so moderation is key.

Tea Time

It's also important not to overlook the option of drinking tea, as it can be a tasty and terrific substitute for coffee. Due to various compounds in tea, its consumption has been linked to numerous heart and health benefits. Specifically, it's been shown that oolong, black, and green teas can help lower the risk of heart disease and high blood pressure, and they can even increase your HDL cholesterol. In fact, a study demonstrated that people who drank oolong or green tea had a 46 to 65 percent decrease in the risk of developing hypertension when compared to non-tea drinkers. While tea's link to cancer prevention has been inconclusive, it's clear that tea has powerful antioxidant and anti-inflammatory properties. Tea has also been tied to an increased level of mental sharpness and alertness, which is ironic given the fact that so many hardworking people cling to coffee for energy instead. Research has also found that drinking tea has been said to aid with weight loss and may reduce the risk of developing type 2 diabetes. But just like with your cup of coffee, if you start adding sugary substances and calorific components, you'll end up adding weight.

ON-THE-GO BREAKFAST

Of course, there are bound to be mornings where things don't go as you'd hoped, but the trick is to have strategies for the unexpected. Just like at work, you need to anticipate and manage unforeseen situations by having contingency plans to match the circumstances. If you receive a frantic email from your boss, need to make a quick change to a presentation, or have to leave early to avoid a traffic jam, there's no need to jam an unhealthy morning meal into your mouth. Come on! Prepare yourself ahead of time for these types of mornings by having portable and on-the-go breakfast foods on hand, especially those that can fit in your hand. Fruits are a fan favorite for an on-the-move breakfast, specifically bananas due to their high potassium level which has been shown to help lower blood pressure, along with the fact that they're naturally prepackaged thanks to their peel.

Yogurt is also a great breakfast pick when you're in a pre-work time pickle, especially since you can choose from a seemingly endless assortment of low-fat and nonfat flavors, types, and textures in single serving sizes—including Greek yogurt which has practically double the amount of protein found in regular yogurt. Along those lines, there are single servings of cottage cheese which are also full of calcium and protein that help you stay fuller longer. An extra benefit of these types of quick morning meals is that research has shown that those who ate low-fat dairy products such as yogurt and cottage cheese actually lowered their risk of developing type 2 diabetes by 24 percent when compared to non-eaters.

Another popular on-the-go option is the breakfast bar, but don't be fooled by the types that could actually double as candy bars, since many bars are merely wolves in sheep's clothing ready to devour your weight loss goals. Nutritionists contend that the trick to tackling the breakfast bar fight is to examine labels and find the options that contain three grams of fiber, five grams of protein, and are low in fat and sugar. It's time for you to be the wolf and separate the right bars from the herd. Even if you face a hectic morning, there's no time to get sheepish when it comes to your weight.

GOING OUT FOR BREAKFAST

Whether they're stopping at a coffee shop or picking up fast food, countless employees are getting breakfast on the way to work each day. And the numbers are there to prove it, both on the scale and otherwise. These ubiquitous eateries can be a major source of weight gain—but only if you allow it to happen. You need to be extremely vigilant when determining your selection. A macchiato and scone can easily hit 600 calories and twenty grams of fat. A blended coffee drink and a morning bun will get you around 700 calories and fifteen grams of fat. And what about your traditional bacon and egg sandwich? Plan on approximately 600 calories and thirty grams of fat. Pancakes and a biscuit can run over 1,000 calories and fifty grams of fat. Obviously, you get the point. And the pounds.

If you still feel compelled to stop at the coffee shops and fast food eateries that line your path to work, the key is to plan ahead. Go online, check the menus, and do everything in your power to unlock the healthiest choices that are offered at your dining destination. There are nutrition guides and guidelines listed on many websites and menus, as well as special sections that list items that fall below a certain calorie count. Plus, you may even find healthier foods and versions of items that you didn't know existed at your eatery of choice. Many of these establishments now serve fruit, yogurt, cottage cheese, oatmeal, as well as lower-calorie and reduced-fat baked goods. In terms of drinks, you can put your own spin on many of them by selecting sugar-free and low-sugar syrups and powders, nonfat milk, and forgoing the whipped cream. Also, keep your size selection in mind. There may be smaller cup sizes that are not widely publicized. You might not know about this option and end up selecting a larger size and ultimately become a larger size yourself. The key to tackling this kind of potential drink deception is to do your research. You do it when making work decisions, and you certainly shouldn't be misinformed when making food decisions. All you have to do is ask.

STAYING IN FOR BREAKFAST

In terms of the bigger picture, you're missing out on a much healthier and cost-effective option if you believe that the only place where you can find these special morning meals is at your preferred eatery. That option is your home. If you're stopping on the way to work to satisfy a breakfast sweet tooth, your supermarket can actually provide you with food choices that make super swap-outs for the crap you're used to ingesting. Look for choices such as low-fat and low-calorie muffins and bagels, as well as whole grain breads which pair nicely with nut butters and sugar-free jellies. You can even venture into the frozen section and find light waffles and pancakes. Speaking of frozen foods, if you're a breakfast sandwich aficionado, you'll find some healthier premade options, some with meat substitutes, that turn your breakfast into a meal that prepares—and not impairs—you to take on the workday and manage your weight. Also, don't overlook making your own egg sandwich with egg whites, low-fat cheese, and whole grain bread. And while there's some debate regarding pork bacon versus turkey bacon in terms of what's "healthier," choose lower salt options and be mindful of the amount of any other processed meats you may be eating throughout the day. The serving size is listed on the package for a reason, so don't go hog wild. You're not irresponsible at work, so don't be reckless in this instance and pig out.

Smooth Moves

Want another figure-friendly and inexpensive breakfast alternative that's a super cool item in the fast food world? Look no further than the do-it-yourself smoothie. A simple online search will unlock a "whirled" of super healthy, easy, and fast smoothie recipes that are superb substitutes for the sugary drinks, blends, and shakes you're used to slurping down. Their ingredients can include fresh and frozen fruits, vegetables, protein powders, tofu, nuts and nut butters, almond milk, soy milk, Greek yogurts, and even coconut water. It can be nothing but smooth(ie) sailing when it comes to your weight if you put in the time—and the right ingredients.

Plug and Chug

If stopping to pick up coffee is how you get your pre-work pick-me-up, it's also time to pick up a calculator. Assume that the average sixteen-ounce fast food cup of coffee costs $2.00. If you buy a cup every weekday, you'll spend approximately $520.00 over the course of a year. However, if you choose to brew your own coffee each workday at home, it'll cost you approximately $95.00 per year. What would you do with the $425.00 that you save? How much of it is already going down the drain? Brewing over buying makes the most sense and cents. Imagine the time you can save in the morning by not having to stop and wait in the long lines at these eateries, whether at a drive-through or inside. Those lines can take forever and a day. You can also eradicate the possibility of human error when it comes to your order, especially during peak and packed morning hours. Plus, by not having to venture to these eateries, you eliminate the possibility of being tempted by all the goodies that grab hold of your senses the moment you arrive. Do the math and lose the mass.

THE PRE-WORK WORKOUT

Many working individuals find it difficult to incorporate a workout routine into their workday routines. Why? Because of their jobs. With jam-packed schedules, long hours, and numerous other tasks and commitments, it seems as though there isn't enough time to incorporate exercise into their busy lives. And as exercise falls by the wayside, sizes and waistlines go way up. But you know that exercise plays a crucial role in any health and weight management program, and that means now's the time to start exercising your right to exercise. Even with your numerous work responsibilities, you still have a responsibility to put yourself first and not let these outside obligations obliterate your workout efforts and the health and wellness benefits they provide. That excuse just doesn't cut it anymore, so move on. Literally, move! With some experimenting, planning, and implementing, you can create a new exercise routine that works.

Exercising Options

One possible strategy to tackle the workday workout challenge is to exercise in the morning before heading off to work. You can go to the gym, or there are many different exercise programs and classes such as spinning, Bikram yoga, and strength training that have early-morning hours that cater to working people.

However, you don't need expensive memberships or fancy equipment to get your heart rate up. The key to exercising—and sticking with it—is to find an activity that you enjoy and will feel inspired to continue. Aside from run-of-the-mill treadmills and ellipticals, channel the creativity you use on your job and find an activity that you like, whether it's walking outside, following a yoga DVD, watching an online Pilates video, or even blasting your favorite pump up songs and dancing around your bedroom. Experts contend that 150 minutes of exercise per week is an appropriate goal, and research in *Applied Physiology, Nutrition, and Metabolism* revealed that racking up those minutes is actually more important than the frequency of how often you work out. Specifically, a study looked at 2,324 Canadian adults who divided up their 150 minutes of exercise into five to seven sessions per week versus one to four times per week. Surprisingly, both groups' risk for hypertension, high cholesterol, high blood sugar, and obesity remained about the same. The takeaway from this study is that workouts can be tailored to any schedule and still generate a wide range of positive outcomes.

A Matter of Timing

And then there's the question of when to eat breakfast if your pre-work morning consists of a workout. The truth is that this issue has been debated for years. Some studies have shown that exercising before breakfast may be more effective at burning fat than exercising after eating since your body will draw on stored energy from fat as opposed to sugar from a recent meal. This makes it a popular choice for those seeking weight loss. Other research has claimed that the amount of fat you burn is fairly consistent whether or not you eat, and you may even end up losing muscle instead. Further, in terms of improving physical fitness, exercising without eating beforehand may also lessen the amount of energy you're able to exert during your workout because you have less fuel in your system. While it's clear there's some dispute regarding breakfast and workouts, it really comes down to what works best for you and your body. If you tend to feel sluggish, tired, and famished when you don't eat before a workout, then obviously eat. A lot of people choose a happy compromise by having a pre-workout morning snack, especially since it's recommended that you give your body time after eating a meal—some say at least forty-five minutes—before working out. Whether you have whole grain toast with almond butter and sliced banana, a banana smoothie, or simply a banana, experimenting will help you find the food type, amount, and timing beforehand that'll get you through your workout. But whether you choose to have breakfast pre-workout or not, drinking water before, after, and even during your workout is crucial in terms of staying hydrated. It's also recommended that you eat within two hours post-workout to help your body recover, especially a snack or a meal that contains combinations of both protein and carbs such as Greek yogurt with fruit or chicken with sweet potato.

Chapter 3

Taking the Weight Out of Your Commute

Your commute to and from work is a key component of your job, bookending your physical presence at the workplace each day. At the same time, unless you're walking or pedaling each way, your commute is going to do a real job on your waistline.

Granted there are several options you can select when it comes to commuting, census data indicate that 86.1 percent of all workers commute by car, truck, or van, and 76.1 percent make these journeys alone. And if you're among the 5 percent who take buses, subways, and trains to work, you'll soon see that these means of transportation don't necessarily free you from the waist enhancement associated with commuting. By and large, the only commuters who are not subject to commuter corpulence are those who either ride a bike or walk, and that's a whopping 3.5 percent, made up of 2.9 percent walkers and .6 percent bikers. So unless you bike it or hike it, you're likely to be putting on the pounds while putting on the miles. And if you're part of the huge percentage of workers who drive or are driven to and from work, the reality is that your commute is a major driver of weight gain.

WHETHER YOU'RE A DRIVER OR A PASSENGER

If an automobile is your means of transportation to and from work, especially if you're behind the wheel, but even if you're riding shotgun or in the backseat, you've no doubt experienced the dent that commuting can put on your mood, emotions, performance, and productivity. Walk into your office after a tough ride to work and you're likely to need more than a few minutes to set the madness of the motorway aside, switch your mindset from warrior to worker, and redirect your attention to the workload that awaits.

Commuting and Your Wellness

However, the physical and mental strains associated with your commute don't end when you step out of the car. Rather, research is finding that commuting is linked to myriad health problems, with many studies showing a compelling relationship between commuting and high cholesterol, high blood sugar, and heart disease. Although these conditions are typically more pronounced as commuting time increases, they're not confined to legendary long treks—they can easily emanate from commutes that are relatively short and arguably mild. Just to get a little perspective, census data indicate that the average commute is approximately twenty-five minutes. Is that a long ride or a short one? If you consider the fact that it translates to more than four full days in the car each year, even the average commute sounds painfully protracted.

Commuting and Your Waist

Research findings regarding commuting and weight gain are nothing short of compelling. Some of these studies specifically call out the automobile as the culprit, as illustrated by a major 2013 study in Australia. Of 822 participants, those who commuted to work by car on a daily basis gained more weight than those who used other means to get to and from their jobs, including buses, bicycles, and trains. This study also found that weight gain associated with driving even occurred for those participants who maintained a good deal of physical activity during their non-work hours. Among the participants who exercised at least two-and-a-half hours a week, those who commuted daily to work in cars still gained more weight than those who used other means of commuting or worked from their homes. In other words, weight gain associated with driving to work is not mitigated by a high degree of physical activity during your non-work hours. In fact, in this study, the only participants who didn't gain weight were those who exercised regularly during the week and didn't commute to work by car.

Similar results were found in a study conducted by public sciences health researchers at Washington University in St. Louis. In analyzing 4,300 commuters in Dallas, Fort Worth, and Austin, it was found that longer car commutes were correlated not only with high blood pressure and other factors that contribute to the likelihood of chronic disease, but also with increases in body mass, belly fat, waist size, and obesity. In this regard, approximately 18 percent of commuters with rides of less than fifteen minutes were obese, while over 25 percent of the commuters whose drives were more than fifteen miles were obese.

At the same time, commuters in buses, subways, and trains don't necessarily disembark from these conveyances with a clean bill of health. A Swedish study with more than 21,000 participants aged eighteen to sixty-five found unhealthy outcomes associated with these seemingly healthier transportation options—certainly when compared with walking or biking to and from work. In most instances, the longer the participants' commutes, whether by car, subway, or bus, the more they voiced health-related complaints. The means of transportation to and from work were not the issue. Rather, the overall focal point was the relationship between the length of the commute and decreased feelings of wellness.

The bottom line is that it's time to take a hard look at your commute and its role in your weight gain. While the problems associated with commuting are indeed serious, they aren't insurmountable. You may be a commuter, but this doesn't necessarily mean that you're sentenced to ongoing health issues and weight gain. Fortunately, to the extent that such a sentence exists, it can be commuted. All it takes is an understanding of the actual causes behind commuting and corpulence, and then establishing and following an action plan to prevent them from tipping the scales against you.

LOOKING BEHIND COMMUTING AND WEIGHT GAIN

If you were somehow asked to develop a system that's all but certain to cause weight gain among its users, you'd be hard-pressed to come up with something more effective than today's commutes. They're uniquely structured to place an individual in a situation in which several of the most powerful fattening forces all come together to build body mass.

Prolonged Sitting

The most obvious reason why commuting plays a central part in weight gain is that it's a prolonged sedentary activity, especially if you ride by car or vanpool. Even if you take public transportation, you may be sitting for extended amounts of time. There's no question that protracted sitting is one of the worst things you can do for your well-being, as it's not only linked to obesity, but also to problems associated with mental health, heart disease, and even a greater likelihood of being disabled.

Reduced Time for Other Pursuits

Not only is your long and sedentary commute taking a toll on your body, it's taking a toll on the time that you have for other activities, many of which would do wonders for your weight and overall health. Using data from the 24,861 full-time employees who participated in the American Time Use Survey, researchers at Brown University found that people who spend an hour each day in their commute—a chunk of time that's very close to today's average round trip—end up with 28 to 35 percent less time for sleeping, 16.1 percent less time for going to the gym or exercising, and 4.1 percent less time for food preparation. And with longer commutes, the numbers are even worse. Sleeping, exercising, and healthy food preparation all play key roles in maintaining physical health and weight control, and today's commute is eating away at each of them.

Stressors and Commuters

There's a strong relationship between stress and weight gain, and your daily commute drives you into an unending stream of stressors. In a 2014 Nielsen survey, two factors tied for first when it comes to causing stress on the job—low pay and long commutes. If you're behind the wheel, some of the stressors include traffic, detours, potholes, crazy drivers, accidents, near-accidents, broken signals, horrible weather, and car problems. If you're a carpool passenger, there can be stress associated with late pick-ups, irritating fellow carpoolers, dangerous or nauseating driving, loud music, and endless boring conversations. If you commute by subway, train, or bus, you too are subjected to an ongoing bar-rage of stressors, such as delays, pushing and shoving, unwanted closeness of fellow riders, malodorous co-riders, nauseating food odors, unwanted physical contact, loud noises, unsolicited solic-itations, claustrophobia, unanticipated stops and starts, subway dust, and more.

Once any of these stressors hit your radar screen, one clear message from your brain is for you to flip into food consumption mode—preferably for so-called comfort foods such as candy, cookies, donuts, and other sweet savories. These foods set you up for the only rush you're likely to see on your commute, namely a sugar rush, followed by a crash—a sugar crash. This certainly gives a whole new meaning to the notion of rush hour.

Slow Commutes and Fast Food

Another important related finding is that longer commutes increase the likelihood that you'll purchase fast food. Whether it's stress, boredom, habit, the power of suggestion, the quest for comfort food, the lack of time to go to the supermarket and pre-pare a healthy meal, a futile attempt to regain some of the time that was lost in travel, a desire to be in a line that moves quicker than most traffic, quasi-instant gratification, superficial social interaction, or stress-induced cravings, fast food offers a broad range of reinforcement for weary road warriors who have been sapped and zapped by their commutes.

For many commuters, making a pit stop for fast food is an everyday occurrence on the way to and from work. Because of the short-term satisfaction associated with this behavior, it can easily become a deeply ingrained habit. On a rational level, most of these partakers know that what they're consuming is not good for them, but such consumption gives them short-term pleasure, and that's enough reinforcement for them to hit the drive-through line. After all, nothing else about their commute is particularly satisfying, and surely they deserve some sort of reward for enduring the travel travails each day. Ultimately, these commuters become dependent on their fast food fix, and going without it can lead to moodiness, angst, and distress. After getting their fix, many will even rationalize that they'll walk it off, but unfortunately, their long commutes have eaten up a chunk of the time to do so. As a result, these commuters end up eating a potpourri of fat, sugar, and calories, all of which will ride with them long after their commutes have ended.

EXERCISE IN MOTION

Fortunately, no matter how you commute to and from work, there are steps you can take along the way that'll make your trek a less fattening and caloric trip. These steps can be as major as you'd like. Take a look at the range of options, experiment with any that appeal to you, and then incorporate those that work as you go to and from work. Whether you're in the driver's seat or the passenger seat, there are light exercises that can help you keep your muscles toned and taut. This is not a cardio workout, but a car workout. You're probably not going to bulk up while buckled up, but you're going to counteract the potential weight gain that comes from sitting around while driving around.

Exercising in Cars

Looking first at the 86.1 percent of commuters who go to and from work by car and carpool, whether as drivers, passengers, or both, there are some easy ways to make your sojourn less of an obesity odyssey, starting with some low-impact exercises. While the realities of the road and the confines of the car certainly eliminate the possibility of jumping jacks and push-ups, you may be surprised to find that there are many highly effective exercises that fit perfectly into your seat. At the same time, safety comes first when engaging in these mobile calisthenics. If you're the driver, most of them are best used when stopped in traffic or at a red light.

Since commuting takes a daily bite out of the time that you can allocate to exercise, here's a way to get some of that time back. The idea is that as you sit in your car, you have an average of an hour per day to vegetate or use a block of that time to tone up some of your muscles, counteract some of the damage associated with sitting inertly for extended periods of time, experience less fatigue, burn up a few calories, reduce your stress levels, make your commute feel shorter, lower your level of boredom, and thereby redirect your focus and interest away from food intake, especially for comfort foods.

Heads Up

The exercises are easy to remember, since they run from head to toe. Starting with your head, just think about nodding "yes" or "no." You probably do this already, such as when you nod your head in glee as the jackass who cut you off gets pulled over by the highway patrol. When you see a reckless or enraged driver, you just might shake your head in annoyance, disgust, or pity. Since you know that you can safely engage in these motions in reaction to the absurd antics of other drivers, why wait for them before making this exercise a regular part of your drive? While keeping your eyes on the road, you can easily do ten "yes" nods, followed by ten "no" nods, and then repeat this set up to five times. A similar exercise is to slowly lean your head to the right and hold it for two seconds, and then lean it to the left and hold it for two seconds. As the driver with your eyes peeled on the road, you'd repeat this set up to five times.

Shouldering the Load

The next stop is your shoulders, and one easy exercise in this area involves pushing your shoulder blades forward, holding them in that position for five to ten seconds, bringing them back and relaxing, and then repeating for ten reps. A related exercise is the simple motion of moving your shoulders up and down, also known as shrugging. It's another move that you can easily do while driving, and it's one of the therapeutic exercises recommended to build shoulder strength. Go with ten shrugs, followed by a few deep breaths, up to a total of five sets.

By the way, there's a psychological side to these shrugs that's also quite appealing. When people shrug, they rarely do so in anger or on impulse. Rather, it's a preplanned low-key response that typically indicates that you either don't know or care about a particular matter. By shrugging when you're driving or riding in a car, the subtle message that you're sending to yourself is that whatever is distressing you on the road is simply not all that important. Your shrug helps you shrug off some of the stressors on the streets.

Back to Work

Just down the road from your shoulders is your lower back. One of the most effective stretches in this area is called the pelvic tilt, and it's easily done while sitting. All you need to do is push your hips forward and feel the small of your back pushing against the back of the seat. The idea is to make the tilt, hold it for five seconds, relax for five seconds, and then repeat this motion ten times.

Stomaching the Ride

If you take a quick spin around the corner from your lower back, you'll arrive at your stomach. This is an area that's particularly susceptible to the expansion, widening, and softening associated with prolonged sitting. Fortunately, the exercises that help reduce wiggling and jiggling in this area are easy to stomach, and they can be practiced when moving or stalled. One approach is to inhale and pull in your stomach as far as you can, hold it for a few seconds, release and exhale. Along with five to ten reps of this breathtaking exercise, a related strategy is to simply tighten your stomach muscles, hold them and count to ten, release and exhale, and then go with five to ten sets. Will these exercises guarantee a flat belly? Nope. But they can help a fat belly.

Handy Exercises

Your arms and hands have a role to play as you roll along. If you're in the driver's seat, these are exercises to consider only when you're totally stopped. Whether you're a driver holding the wheel or a passenger holding a conversation, one way to help prevent your arms from becoming flabby is to make a fist and tighten your arm muscles, hold this for a few seconds, release, relax, and repeat. A related exercise is to place one hand in front of you and then open and close it fifty times. When you finish with one hand, do the same thing with the other. This leads to further toning of your hand muscles and forearms.

For passengers only, you can do more with your arms by repeatedly lifting them toward the ceiling. Think of yourself as doing a mini-dance and raising the roof. If you want to take the roof-raising idea a little further, you can even bring a couple of light weights along for the ride and use them during this phase of your road work. Another exercise just for passengers entails using hand grips—small hand-sized devices—that offer resistance as you squeeze them. It's a great way to pass the time and strengthen your hands and forearms. Plus, when you're holding hand grips, you're less likely to be holding anything else, such as a donut or muffin.

As part of this program, there are exercises for drivers only which involve the use of the steering wheel. If you're driving and find yourself at a standstill, place both hands securely on opposite sides of the wheel and push as if you're attempting to turn the round wheel into an oval. Do this for five seconds, relax, and then do ten more reps. A variation is to pull your hands in opposite directions as if you're stretching out the wheel, following the same program with five seconds of pulling and relaxing.

Rear View

The next exercise focal point is your rear—namely your glutes. One of the best exercises to avoid the flabbiness and sagginess associated with prolonged sitting is to tighten the butt muscles, hold for a count of five or ten, relax, and follow with five more sets. In order to achieve maximum safety while tightening your gluteus maximus, this is another exercise that should be done when you're totally stopped if you're behind the wheel. As you sit and cogitate the congestion, this exercise is likely to come to mind, since you're instantly reminded that commuting is a pain in the butt.

Leg of Your Journey

There are some particularly effective leg exercises for passengers. Start by tightening the muscles in your upper leg, hold for ten seconds, relax, and then repeat this set five to ten times. This is followed by using the exact same steps with your calf muscles. As an easy way to remind yourself of this exercise, when you're in gridlock, think of a leg-lock. A related exercise is to lift your legs, one at a time, a few inches from the floor, tightening your thigh, and holding each leg up for five seconds. You'd do this with one leg and then the other for five reps. This exercise helps you get a leg up on the problems associated with extended sitting and weight gain.

A Feat with Your Feet

Another exercise for passengers only is to plant your heel on the floor and then raise the rest of your foot and hold it for ten seconds, drop it down, and then alternate from one foot to the other. You can also do the opposite of this exercise, namely by planting your toes on the floor, lifting your heels, holding for ten seconds, dropping them down, and then repeating while you again alternate from one foot to the other. For a little more strengthening, try doing these exercises with your briefcase, purse, or both on your lap. Also just for passengers, one excellent range-of-motion exercise that's used for all sorts of foot and ankle ailments is to spell the alphabet with each foot. Think of each foot as a pen, and your goal is to use that pen to slowly write out the alphabet, one letter at a time.

There are even exercises for your toes, and it simply entails wiggling them. You can scrunch them up, flare them apart, bend them upward or downward, and just keep them moving. It's not as if this exercise is going to condition any of your little piggies to the point that you'll run all the way home, but it does work in combination with the previous exercises to help you make and take the most out of your ride to and from work.

EXERCISING IN BUSES AND TRAINS

If you're among the 5 percent of commuters who ride to and from work in buses, trains, and subways, you too may find yourself sitting for extended periods of time and subjecting yourself to commuter corpulence. Fortunately, these forms of transportation offer a number of opportunities to exercise along the way. Just for starters, if your ride includes a good deal of sitting, you can use the same exercises as passengers in cars.

If you're riding on these conveyances, you don't have to sit at all. Sometimes, you won't even be able to find a seat, and that's not such a bad outcome. In fact, you should actually try to stand— and take a stand against weight gain. By doing so, you can engage in any number of stand-up stretching exercises and even get in some cardio before and after work.

Hold It!

If you're on a bus or train and determine that conditions are safe, you can stand and hold onto the pole, handrail, or strap for stability and safety. Once you're up, you can continue the stretching that you were doing while sitting, such as flexing your stomach, shrugging your shoulders, and turning your head from one direction to the other. When you're standing, many exercises work even better. You can easily extend one arm and then the other to the ceiling, and this is a great way to build your abs, biceps, and triceps, while also enhancing your overall strength and endurance. These reaches work particularly well if you're lifting some weight, whether you're holding small dumbbells or wearing wrist weights. Reach for the sky with one hand ten times, bring your hand to your side, take a deep breath, and do the same series with the other hand.

Another safe and easy exercise while standing and holding on during your commute on a bus or train is to stand on your tiptoes, hold for ten seconds, slowly let your heels down, and then repeat. This can do wonders for your calves while stretching your Achilles tendons as well. And going a step further, you can even hold onto the handrail or pole and slowly lift one knee, keep it elevated for ten seconds, and then repeat with the other leg.

DE-STRESSING YOUR COMMUTE

With commuting consistently noted as one of the greatest sources of job-related stress, in combination with the fact that increases in stress lead to increases in appetite, especially for foods that are low on the nutritious scale and high on the bathroom scale, managing the stress of your commute ends up being one of your most important managerial responsibilities—whether you're a manager or not. The good news is that exercising while commuting can also help you reduce stress on the road, especially when combined with other proven stress management techniques.

Breathe Easy

Whether by car, bus, or train, one of the best ways to handle whatever is stressing you out in your commute is deep breathing. As you feel yourself tensing up, slowly inhale through your nose, hold your breath for a few seconds, and then slowly exhale through your mouth. By repeating this a few times, you can start to turn the stress levels down and better cope with the stress of the road or rails.

A Sound Decision

Another way to soften the impact of commuter stress is with soft music on your radio, smartphone, or headset, especially some peaceful classical pieces. In terms of music's effectiveness in calming you down, many studies have found that classical music is strongly associated with reductions of stress, anxiety, and negativity. In fact, in one classic study, classical music was found to be more effective in reducing anxiety than anti-anxiety meds for preoperative and postoperative patients. Further, by coordinating your exercise with this music, you can compound their stress-reducing powers. This should be music to your ears.

You can also access other stress-reducing audio offerings while you're commuting, such as entertaining novels, podcasts, or satellite radio programs. In addition, you can listen to specifically designed stress-reducing tutorials that can help increase relaxation, renewal, and mindfulness during a crazy commute. And if you're a passenger, you have a wider range of options to help manage your stress—reading, watching your favorite shows or movies, and texting with friends.

Pre-Commute Planning

The stress of your commute can also be diminished by doing some advance planning. Since planning is inherent in virtually every job, it should be equally inherent in virtually every commute. One of the major stressors in a commute is the anxiety associated with arriving late to work. A train is delayed, a traffic light is broken, an accident occurs ahead—it seems that there's something every day that interferes with your timely commute and your state of mind. And yet, there are methods to head off this stress before it gets into your head. The most obvious is to leave for work a little earlier. Granted there may be other early morning commitments such as with children's schools that make this more difficult, many schools have programs to accommodate commuter needs. For the sake of your health and your waistline, such options are worth exploring.

Also on the planning front, be sure to look ahead at the route that you'll be taking by using apps and websites that provide real-time information on traffic, accidents, road conditions and hazards, and optimum routes. Whether you're driving all the way to work or just to the subway station or park-and-ride lot, selecting the routes that flow the best will do wonders in easing your commute and reducing the stress associated with it.

More De-Stressing Ideas

There's a potpourri of additional actions to further reduce the stress that accompanies your ride to and from work. Studies have found that using a seat cushion is an excellent way to lessen the stress of a long commute. Another way to make your ride more tolerable is to reduce some of the stressors associated with your car or van. If there are loose items such as empty plastic bottles that are rolling around and annoying you at every turn, toss them into a recycling bin. If the windshield is so filled with dirt, dust, and bird droppings that you're squinting through the smudges to see the road, take a grand total of thirty seconds and clean it. Further offerings in this stress-deflating package include smiling, singing, and even sniffing pleasant aromas. Researchers at Wheeling Jesuit University found that smelling peppermint and cinnamon while driving led to higher levels of alertness while reducing frustration and fatigue. Aromatherapy while commuting—not a bad idea if your commute stinks.

COMMUTING AND CONSUMING

If you're like most of today's commuters, the mere act of getting into a car, whether as a driver or a passenger, can set your salivary glands in motion. No, you're not salivating over the ride, but over the prospect of munching and crunching along the way. Even if you drive alone, you're not dining alone. In a study of 1,000 drivers conducted by ExxonMobil, over 70 percent admitted that they eat while driving.

There can be any number of reasons behind this phenomenon. For some drivers, the desire to toss down some food comes as a result of sheer boredom. They drive the same old route every day, to the point that they even see some of the same drivers on the road. In order to break this monotony and throw some spice and variety into the drive, they reach for a bag of goodies. Then there are the eaters who are driven to snack out of a need to reduce stress. Related to this stress reaction, some people will eat while driving because they sense that they deserve a reward or prize for putting up with the insanity on the interstate. With this mindset, it's not as if they're eating for the sake of eating, but rather as a form of personal gratification and recognition for navigating the treachery of the traffic.

There's also a cadre of mobile eaters who use the ride to and from work as a time to eat their meals. Some of these commuters bring food from home, while others break up their drive with a quick visit to an eatery along the way. For others, the respite at the fast food eatery is for food and more, as there's a social gratification associated with seeing the same people each day, schmoozing with them, and then saying goodbyes and heading off in all directions. If your commute has become a moveable feast of fatty foods, you're tossing your weight control plan out the power window.

Putting on the Brakes

If your commuting snacks are cookies, cupcakes, muffins, candies, or any other consumables of the high-caloric, high-sugar, and high-fat variety, it's time to stop driving your weight management plan and goals into the ground. You can easily plan ahead and replace your car carbs and crap with healthier commuter-friendly offerings. Snacks such as low-fat and low-sugar bars, fruits, and nuts can easily fill the bill and fill you up. Speaking of nuts, they can be extra special for commuters since research indicates they can help reduce stress—especially cashews and walnuts. In addition, you should always have a bottle of water with you. Hydration not only has a positive impact on every system in your body, it also helps counteract the stress and resultant hunger associated with commuting.

If you're a stop-and-snack commuter who likes to hit the fast food outlets, you don't have to eliminate these stopovers from your commute. All you need to do is stop salivating over their fatty and sugary offerings and take a look at the healthy options that many eateries now provide. By planning your selections ahead, you can steer clear of the unhealthy foods that take you and your commute in the wrong direction.

In dealing with these eateries, an additional point to keep in mind is to avoid the drive-through line. From a practical standpoint, there's some debate over how much time this line will actually save you. From the health standpoint, sitting in these lines is just that—sitting. And this is simply compounding your sedentary commute. Rather than sitting idly while your car idles, you should use these pit stops as an opportunity to walk, stretch, and get your cardiovascular system going. You can do this by ignoring the drive-through, parking a good distance from the restaurant, walking to it, and then stretching, bending, and moving in place while waiting in line.

COMMUTING OUTSIDE THE BOX

As you consider your commute's relationship to your food intake and weight gain, there's a wide range of healthy options that can help prevent you from becoming wider. It calls for you to view your commute in a totally different light.

Bike It

The first option is to consider commuting by bicycle. While a great deal depends on the distance of your commute and available roads and bike lanes, there are major advantages associated with commuting by bike. Biking to and from work can help you burn calories, save money that would be spent on gas plus wear and tear on your car, reduce your stress, increase endorphin production, enhance your cardiovascular health, lower your BMI, and generate additional satisfaction by going green. Further, commuting to work by bicycle has been linked to lower absentee rates because of sickness. In a study of 1,236 Dutch employees, the more frequently that the participants cycled to work and the greater the distance that they traveled, the less likely they were to call in sick. If the cost of owning a bike is an issue, there are very affordable bike-share programs cropping up in cities around the world.

Commuter Combo

For many employees, converting your entire commute into a cycling activity might not be feasible. However, other related options might work. There are ways to combine the healthiest commuting practices—cycling, walking, and public transportation—into a mixture that works for you. If you commute to work by car, some of the combo steps that you can take include parking your car a mile or so from work and walking the difference. If this isn't workable, don't fight for that parking spot closest to your workplace. Take the spot on the farthest side of the lot and walk it. And when you get to the building, if you have a choice between the elevator and the stairs, always opt for the stairs.

If a bike ride is too long or impossible because of the required route, you can even combine cycling with driving to work by attaching a bike rack to your car, parking the car a couple of miles from work, and then biking the balance of the distance to and from your job. You can also combine biking with public transportation and gain even more advantages. The idea would be to ride your bike to the bus stop or subway station and bring the bike with you as you embark. If you're taking a bus, most city buses have racks where you can easily stow your bike. Also, many subway systems are now far more receptive to bikes at all hours of the day, while there may be restrictions in loading your bike onto the first few cars. In either of these cases, it's always helpful to check out the transportation provider's website to get a clear understanding of the ground rules. At the same time, if you have a folding bike, you can bring it onboard.

Exercise This

By the way, when you're using public transportation with or without a bike, you can get in some extra exercise in several different ways. Keep moving while you're waiting for the bus or train such as by walking around or walking in place. You can also get off one or two stops before your usual stop and walk the distance as well as take the stairs whenever possible. You should also consider getting off a stop or two early when you bring your bike and then pedal the distance. These walking, biking, and riding permutations are not cast in stone. You can mix them up in any fashion that best suits your needs, such as by driving a couple of days a week, doing the bus and walk combo on another day, carpooling the next day, and so forth as you go forth.

Alternate Rides

You can also take advantage of some of the newer ways to get to and from work. There are many apps that bring drivers directly to you, and some employers have hopped onboard by establishing cost-effective relationships with these services to transport employees to and from work. Some companies also have their own vanpool programs or even their own buses that can facilitate your work commute while removing many of the temptations that can lure you off your weight loss path.

Boredom Busting

If your commuting battle of the bulge is associated with the sheer boredom and tediousness of the trek, one of the most effective ways to combat such ennui is to take a different route to and from work. This would not be a random ride where you expend extra fuel and time, but rather an alternate yet expeditious route, such as one suggested by one of the traffic or map apps. The value of this approach is not merely to introduce a little variety into your ride, but also to break some firmly ingrained behaviors, habits, thought patterns, and conditioning. By taking a different route, you'll see different sights, direct your attention to new focal points, and engage in different physical actions as you navigate your car through the new environs. Right from the get-go, this is guaranteed to be less boring, but there's something deeper at work. When you passed the old familiar sites, they may have generated cues, triggers, and reminders for you to have a snack, often something in the sweet but unhealthy category. Since these stimuli are missing on your new route, the eating response that they prompted will be missing as well.

Management and Your Commute

Another way to control weight gain and your commute is to find out if management in your company would be receptive to flexible hours or telecommuting, even if it's just for a day or two a week. With more variability in your onsite hours, your commute could be moved away from the peak traffic times, thereby allowing you to spend less time in transit. Plus, working from home would eliminate the commute altogether. Either way, the more miles you take off your commute, the more inches you're likely to take off your waist.

AT THE END OF THE JOURNEY

One final piece of business deals with the overarching issue of driving and eating. As you consider the cornucopia of options associated with consuming while commuting, step back and recognize one critical point—if you're behind the wheel and eating, you're significantly increasing your chances of having an accident. In a study conducted by the National Highway Traffic Safety Administration and the Virginia Tech Transportation Institute, it was estimated that approximately 80 percent of accidents involved some aspect of driver distraction. While some of the obvious diversions include texting, phone use, and drowsiness, it's very easy to be a distracted driver when you're reaching around and trying to find a snack, sorting out what you want, fiddling with the wrapper, and picking up whatever dropped in your lap or on the floor. As a result, if you're going to be eating and driving, get your food organized and set up before the ride, and be sure to focus on the main attraction and not the distraction.

Looking further at automobile accidents, an interesting development has emanated as a result of the increased girth and body mass of today's drivers. In order to better reflect this change, crash-test dummies are being redesigned and reconfigured to reflect the larger waistlines and butts of current drivers. At present, crash-test dummies weigh around 167 pounds, while the new models will reflect the body measurements of a 270-pound person.

There's no reason for you to resemble this model. When it comes to your job, your weight management plan, your food intake, your activity level and exercise, and your commute, don't be a dummy.

Chapter 4

Becoming Round by Sitting Around

id you ever stop to ponder the percentage of time on your job that you spend on your butt? If not, you just might want to sit down before you read this. Studies in the United States and Europe have found that the average office employee sits between 65 and 75 percent of the time at work. The reasons behind this massive chunk of time spent on one's glutes are fairly obvious. There's less of a need for you to get up. With email, cell phones, texting, teleconferencing, virtual meetings, webinars, online databases, social media, and more, along with the prospect of having a fellow employee or employer who drops off food at your desk, you hardly ever have to get up. Think back to what you did at work today. How much of that activity was spent while you were in a chair? Does this sit well with you? It shouldn't.

SIDE EFFECTS FROM SITTING

While sitting may feel comfortable, relaxing, and soothing, the side effects can be deadly. In the first place, there's a huge body of research which definitively proves that sitting for prolonged periods of time at work is conducive to weight gain. Researchers at the Mayo Clinic set out to learn why some employees gain weight and others don't. In this study, office workers who didn't engage in much regular exercise were all put on the same diet that included approximately 1,000 additional calories beyond their typical consumption pattern, and they were told not to change their exercise patterns. However, by the end of the study, some participants gained weight while others didn't. In order to investigate the cause of this disparity, researchers tracked the participants' movements with motion sensors and found that those who didn't gain weight spent more time moving, walking, and being generally more active. They walked instead of emailing, took the stairs instead of the elevator, and engaged in myriad additional daily activities and pursuits that called for motion and movement. It turned out that the participants who put on the pounds sat on average two hours longer each day than the participants who didn't gain weight. Similar to the findings of other studies in this area, an employee's failure to get up, get active, and get around is clearly linked to weight gain.

Now, perhaps you're saying to yourself, "But I work out regularly, so even if I sit for hours and hours each day, my exercise regimen is going to protect me from weight gain that comes from sitting at work." Or, "I'm a jogger, so this doesn't apply to me." Unfortunately, these beliefs are incorrect. A great deal of research has proven that even if you engage in these types of fitness activities, your prolonged sitting can undo all of the good that comes from them. Whether you're a runner or not, a study from researchers at the University of Texas Southwest Medical Center found that each segment of time that's spent sitting cancels out 8 percent of whatever was gained by running for the same amount of time. This means that if you ran for one hour before work and then came to work and sat for one hour, 8 percent of the health benefits that you gained from your run disappear. By multiplying this out a little further, if you sit for five hours, you just eliminated 40 percent of your health benefits—and if you sit longer, just do the math and see the benefits go down the drain. By the way, running is regarded as vigorous exercise, and if you engage in exercise that's in the moderate range, you come out even worse—you lose 16 percent of the health benefits you gained.

Inside Information

When you're sitting for prolonged periods, several physiological factors come together to compound your poundage. One major factor is that the mere act of sitting is going to burn far fewer calories than standing, walking, or just about any other activity. Many experts estimate that you can burn at least twenty additional calories per hour just by standing instead of sitting. Further, prolonged sitting slows down your metabolism, and as it slows down, your weight gain speeds up. Sitting also suppresses lipoprotein lipase, an enzyme that removes fat from the blood and transfers it to your muscles to be used during periods of activity. When you're in sitting mode for extended periods of time, less of this enzyme is circulated, and this means that fat is not removed from your blood and absorbed by your muscles. Rather, fat continues to circulate in your bloodstream where it can be stocked up in the form of body fat—further contributing to increased pounds for you. To make matters worse, a number of studies have found that prolonged sitting can lead to an increase in your appetite, which is soon followed by an increase in your weight.

In addition to the compelling link between prolonged sitting and weight gain, research has shown that spending extended periods of time on your derriere is associated with many serious and debilitating physical and mental ailments, including heart disease, high blood pressure, type 2 diabetes, increased levels of LDL cholesterol, various cancers, hypertension, weakened muscles, slower brain function, increased risk of back problems, posture issues, a greater likelihood of becoming disabled, a shortened life expectancy, arthritis, and depression. It's actually depressing to think about what all of this sitting may be doing to you at this very moment.

WHO SAID YOU HAVE TO BE SEDENTARY?

Fortunately, you don't have to take this harrowing news sitting down. You can literally stand up for yourself and do something about it. As is the case with many projects on the job, the first step is to establish some benchmark data by measuring where you are today. This will open your eyes to the current status of the situation, help you establish meaningful and realistic objectives, track and monitor your performance, and provide you with the basis for measurement. Begin by keeping track of two sets of data for a couple of days—one set is how many hours you spend in a chair, and the other is the duration of each sitting spell. You're probably going to be shocked, but that's a good thing, since it's likely to shock you into action.

Initial Steps to Avoid the Scourges of Sitting

When you look at your chair at work, it's time to see it for what it really is—a weight-gaining machine. The more you use it, the more weight you'll gain. Of course you can and should sit some of the time, but the tendency to spend long stretches in your chair is one of the worst things you can do to manage your weight as well as your overall health. As you work your way through the day and carry out your various chores, responsibilities, and tasks, there's one weighty question to repeatedly ask yourself, "Is there a way I could be standing or walking while doing this?" If the answer is yes, do it. On a more subtle basis, by repeating this question to yourself, you're continuously giving yourself a powerful suggestion, "I could be standing or walking while doing this." The more you repeat this, the more this message will sink into your unconscious, and the more likely you'll act on it.

A Moving Experience

One key step in the process is to pay more attention to the duration of your sitting spells. Whenever you find yourself sitting for more than twenty to thirty minutes straight, plan on getting up for a minute or two, doing some light stretching, and then sitting down and going back to work. Will this mini-motion do you any good? Research has proven that even the mildest forms of movement and action play an important role in counteracting the debilitating side effects and wide effects that are associated with protracted sitting.

Standing Phone Calls

The next time your phone rings, you know how tempting it is to pick it up, sit back, relax, and engage in a dialogue. But couldn't you be walking at the same time? You don't need to do push-ups, jumping jacks, or sit-ups during the call. The mere act of standing up and walking around as you speak is all that's necessary, even if it's a brief call. An easy way to remember this is when you think of calls, think of calories, or even better, "call-ories." Whether long or short, these calls add up during the day, and they can all be subtracted from the total time that you spend in sitting mode. You're a stand-up person, and that's exactly what and who you should be when the phone rings.

If you continue to shift into stand-up mode when you hear the phone ring, don't be surprised if you develop a conditioned response in which the sound of a phone causes your brain to automatically send a message for you to rise. When Pavlov's dogs heard the bells ring, they would salivate. When you hear your phone ring, you'll elevate.

Standing Visits

How about when coworkers pop by and plop into a chair for a nice sit-down conversation with you? If you're interested in keeping your life long and these encounters short, you should stand up as soon as they show up. By doing so, you're simultaneously taking many positive steps. First, you're helping your health by getting out of your chair and standing up. The calories start burning immediately. Secondly, when your visitors see that you're standing, they're not likely to sit down, so you're helping them avoid treacheries of sitting. Further, your body language is also telling the visitors that you're busy, and this sends a message for them to cut to the chase and keep their comments focused and on target. People are far more likely to engage in longer conversations if they sit down and get comfortable. Standing up avoids those long rambling discourses that burn time, but not calories. In a more traditional sense, standing up when others enter your office is a sign of respect, and there are some associates, especially individuals in positions higher than yours, who may consciously or unconsciously appreciate this gesture. And so will your waistline.

Standing Meetings

You should apply this same strategy to the meetings you attend, whether you're an organizer or an attendee. As the organizer, one approach is to conduct a basic meeting—ideally in the most remote conference room to add to your walking—and include stretch breaks every twenty to thirty minutes. Physically, this is a way to burn a few calories in the course of the meeting, but there are other businesslike advantages associated with these breaks as well. When the attendees stand up, it's as if they're hitting their restart buttons, and they typically return to the discussion refreshed and even with a new perspective for dealing with the issues at hand.

If you're an attendee in a meeting and find that you have been sitting for more than thirty minutes, you should consider taking your own stand-and-stretch break. Obviously, doing so depends in part on the culture of your organization and the style of the individual who's running the meeting. If you're uncertain as to how this will play out, you can mention to the organizer ahead of time that you may want to stand up and stretch for a minute or two during the meeting if it's okay with her. The response is likely to be positive, along with a question as to why you want to do so. If you mention the potential advantages that can accrue to the meeting as well as to the attendees, you just might find that the organizer includes these breaks on the agenda.

The next step is to take the full plunge and turn traditional meetings into standing or even walking meetings. Such meetings are being held in numerous companies already, and the advantages abound. From the standpoint of weight management, they burn up calories galore. Plus, a study at the Olin Business School at Washington University in St. Louis found that meetings in which the attendees were standing generated a number of positive behaviors, such as increases in enthusiasm and excitement about the work along with reductions in territoriality, all of which led to improved performance of the group itself. But that's just standing meetings. In a series of experiments at the Stanford Graduate School of Education, researchers found that the vast majority of participants consistently demonstrated significantly higher levels of creativity when walking as opposed to sitting. And further, enhanced creative thinking continued for those who returned to sitting soon after walking. If you're wondering if these walking meetings should be indoors or outdoors, the Stanford study found that the setting of the walking had no impact on creativity levels. It was the act of walking that made the difference. As a result, when the objectives of your meeting are focused on coming up with new ideas, solving problems, and general brainstorming, walking meetings are the way to go in every respect. They're a creative and productive way to help manage your weight while managing much more.

More Moving Opportunities

By building your sensitivity and awareness to situations in which you could be moving rather than stationary, you'll easily see that opportunities abound. If you usually ride an elevator or escalator to get to your office or work area, try the stairs. If your office is on the fortieth floor, how about starting with a few flights and working your way up? Also, if you want to enhance the impact of your stair climbing, try going up two stairs at a time. Then there's the email that you're going to send to an associate just down the hall. It's a quick FYI and certainly nothing that needs to be documented. Ditch the email and walk over for a brief stand-up visit with him. This also applies to communicating with coworkers in the office by phone. Rather than picking up your phone, pick up your feet, walk over to your associate, and meet in person. As a side note, when it comes to two-way communication, face-to-face interaction is far more effective than email or even the telephone. When you meet in person, you have the advantage of picking up all sorts of nonverbal cues that help you understand if your message is truly being received. Experts have found that approximately 80 percent of communication is based on non-verbal messages, and those messages fall short of the mark in email and phone conversations.

Water Works

As you know, drinking water during the day is an important component of a weight management plan. Water makes you feel fuller, has no calories, energizes your muscles, balances your body's fluids, and helps your organs function properly. What's less obvious is that water can also contribute to your walking time. First, don't keep a stash of water in your desk or even in your work area. When you feel thirsty, take a hike down the hall to the break room or go upstairs to another work area to fill up your glass or bottle. A less obvious fact that's related to your water consumption is that after you drink, there will come a time when you'll need to pay a visit to the restroom. When nature calls, your "number one" priority shouldn't be to head for the closest lavatory—rather, head for the one that's way down the hall or on another floor.

Copying, Printing, and Walking

Printing and copying also present an opportunity for you to stretch your legs and more. Instead of using the printer on your desk or in your work area, send documents to a printer on the other side of the building or even on a different floor if possible. After you hit print, walk over and retrieve the documents. If they're on another floor, be sure to take the stairs. This same approach applies to making copies. And further, rather than walking to retrieve or copy a batch of papers, break the batch into smaller amounts, print or copy them separately, and then make separate trips to the printer or copier. Isn't this inefficient and wasting time? Not at all. Actually, by doing extra walking, you're going to be saving time since you're likely to be more reenergized when you return to your desk, more likely to engage in innovative thinking that accompanies walking, more likely to gain a fresh perspective that comes from stepping away from your work and then returning to it, and even more likely to miss less work because of illness. Do you copy? By the way, while the printer is printing and the copier is copying, you should be stretching or moving in place.

Trash Talk

As you do your work, you probably accumulate papers and other items that can be recycled, as well as other stuff that simply needs to be tossed. On the one hand, it's easy to have a trash container under your desk or right next to it, and you may even have separate containers for recyclables and non-recyclables. When you need to throw something out, it's only natural to lean over, make your deposit, and then get back to work. By doing so, your energy expenditure and caloric burn are close to zero. But the need to dispose of some trash also poses a potential situation in which you can do some extra walking. Rather than tossing trash into the containers under your desk, take those throwaways to other areas where trash cans are located, preferably in departments or areas that are a reasonable walking distance from yours.

Park and Walk

There's also the matter of your parking place. In many companies, the so-called better spaces are typically closest to the building entrance, elevator, or shuttle. They're usually assigned on the basis of job title, with the more senior-level employees receiving the spots that are closest to those points. Occasionally, an employee-of-the-month is temporarily rewarded with one of these spots. While you may aspire to be employee-of-the-month, you shouldn't aspire to have any of these parking spaces. If you have one now, you should seriously consider a reassignment.

Is It Any Wander?

If you're a manager, you'll definitely want to engage in the well-established practice of managing by wandering around. As the name implies, this calls for managers to get out of their offices, get onto the floors, and make themselves more visible, accessible, and responsive to their employees. By doing so, managers are able to take advantage of one of the most powerful ways to effectively lead a team, namely by managing with all of their senses. By using this information as the basis for ongoing feedback, guidance, and two-way communication, managers are in a far better position to generate increased levels of productivity, satisfaction, and commitment from their team. At the same time, the less obvious advantage of managing by wandering around is centered on the word "wandering." If you're a manager, this strategy automatically implies that you're walking, burning calories, and helping control your weight. Hence, managing by wandering around not only means managing your team, but managing your waistline.

WORKING OUT WHILE WORKING AT YOUR DESK

Although it's apparent that there are many productive ways to significantly increase the time you spend standing and walking on the job, there'll obviously be chunks of time when you'll need to be planted at your desk, chipping away at one project or another. While there's no question that such work should be hyphenated by getting up and around, does this mean that you should you sit passively doing deskwork the rest of the time? Absolutely not. You can definitely do some stretching during those stretches of work, and a lot more.

Up on Arrival

When you arrive at your office or workstation, possibly after walking across the parking lot from the farthest possible spot, hiking up three flights of stairs, and putting away your lunch if you brought one, you'll reach your desk and presumably sit down. However, instead of plopping into your chair, look at this as an exercise opportunity. Stop and stand in front of your chair as if you're going to sit down, but do it very slowly. Gradually lower your torso into the chair, while keeping your spine straight, your stomach firm, your shoulders relaxed, and your arms gently balancing you. Once you're sitting, you're probably going to reach over and boot up your computer. While it's doing so, stand up and do this sitting maneuver a few more times.

Leg It Up

You can also take advantage of some leg exercises while sitting and working at your desk. One way to burn up calories and tone up leg muscles while deskbound is to push your chair back a little, sit with both feet on the floor, and then lift your legs and extend your feet, one leg at a time, hold each fully extended and parallel to the floor for five to ten seconds, and then slowly bring them back to the floor. These reps are a nice way to kick-start your exercise regime while continuing your work at a healthy pace.

Touchdown!

When you're deeply contemplating a perplexing work problem, with your hands resting motionlessly atop your keyboard, calculator, or desk, it's a perfect opportunity to strengthen your arms and shoulders and spin off a few calories by signaling for a touchdown. Thus, as you contemplate the conundrum, continuously raise your arms up and down signaling touchdown after touchdown until you have scored thirty of them. Since this is likely to be a different kind of activity for you, it just might open the door to a different kind of thinking as well, perhaps bringing you a step closer to the end zone.

Sit-and-Run

You can also get in some deskbound exercise by running in place while sitting and working at your desk. Just raise your heels and push off the balls of your feet, lifting your feet a couple of inches each time as you patter away. This little maneuver can burn up a chunk of energy and calories, while strengthening your thighs, calves, ankles, and more. With five minutes of running in place, you're likely to find yourself in a better place.

Tight Situations

Whether finances are tight in your company or not, as you sit and work at your desk, there's some tightening you can do that pays handsome dividends. It begins with inhaling, tightening your glutes, holding for thirty seconds, relaxing, and then exhaling. This is followed by doing the same routine for your stomach, thighs, calves, arms, and fists. Of course, if you're using your keyboard, it's best to clench your fists when you're in mental mode rather than manual mode.

It's a Stretch

Whether your company is trying to stretch dollars or not, there's some stretching that can be very profitable for you as well. When sitting and working at your desk, one great stretch is to lock your fingers as if in prayer, bend them backwards and extend your arms directly in front of you or over your head, and then hold for a count of ten, repeating a few more times. Next, as you work away on your project and stop to think of the perfect sentence to craft, design to create, or code to write, an easy stretch is to reach back with both hands and simply hold onto your shoulder blades. If you're really daring and into something a little more strenuous while still being studious, try placing each hand flat on the chair, next to your thighs, fingers pointing outward, and then straighten your arms and push your buttocks out of the seat of the chair. The idea is to hold yourself up for a few seconds and then slowly lower yourself back down. It's literally a push-up in a chair, engaging muscles in your arms, shoulders, stomach, and back, and you can make it even more powerful by lifting your feet off the floor at the same time. With a few reps, as this exercise pushes you up, it's also going to push up the number of calories you burn.

Other stretches while seated and working at your desk include the neck stretch in which you lean your head to your left shoulder and then over to your right shoulder, holding for ten seconds with each tilt for up to ten reps. You can also stretch your neck muscles by nodding your head in agreement and shaking it in disagreement. If you have a swivel chair, you can get in some productive back stretching and increase your physical activity level by placing both feet on the floor and swiveling from side to side, all the while with your head facing forward and your eyes on your monitor. For a different twist, you can simply twist your torso to the left and right and back again several times, holding at the end of each turn. These are easy to do and easy to remember—just think of the twists and turns that you encounter in your job each day. A little shoulder shrugging is great for the shoulders, and you can easily do it while working. For thigh strengthening, try putting your purse or briefcase between your knees, locking your knees together, and holding them tightly in that position to prevent whatever's between them from falling to the floor. Stay in this position for thirty seconds, grab onto the purse or briefcase for a few seconds, relax your legs, and then repeat. Want to stretch out your lower back? Just push your chair back a few inches and then lean forward as if you're taking a bow. You can do this with your hands on the keyboard and even while you're typing away. With reps of these types of exercises a few times a day, the periods that you spend sitting at your desk will be far less sedentary. By doing these exercises and stretches, you'll be pumping up your heart and metabolism, while simultaneously pumping up your job performance.

IN-BETWEEN MOMENTS

You can also engage in further physical activity in those moments when you need to be in your office or workstation, but not necessarily at your desk. Perhaps you're waiting while a new program is downloading or maybe you have a few minutes of downtime while waiting for an appointment to show up. In these types of scenarios, you not only have the option of stepping away from your desk and doing some standing and walking, but you can also squeeze in some exercises and stretches as well.

Range of Motion

Also during these periods, how about standing in place and doing some light marching or jogging, or even some easy jumping up and down? A minute or two will do. You could knock off a few traditional push-ups on the floor or simply place your arms on the wall and do the standing version. These are calorie burners, and they're good for your biceps, triceps, back, thighs, calves, and shoulder muscles, too. You can also do a slightly different version of this stretch by placing both of your legs farther back, keeping your heels on the floor, and then slowly leaning to the wall and stretching out your calves. You can also do this one leg at a time. Speaking of the wall, one stretch that's great for the lower back is to stand against the wall and tilt your pelvis forward so that the small of your back flattens out. Hold this position for five seconds and repeat. This is excellent for strengthening your back muscles and stomach muscles. Also, with your back against the wall, in a good way, you can do some further strengthening by bending your knees and slowly dropping down until your legs look like you're a baseball catcher. Hold this position for a few seconds and then slowly stand up as your back slides up the wall. An easy way to remember this stretch is that as you do your work, it's always good to have a back-up plan.

Another low-impact exercise that can have a high impact on your calf muscles is simply to stand up with your feet pointed straight ahead, and then go onto your tiptoes, hold for five seconds, drop down, and then repeat. You can also stand in the same position, raise your right leg, grab it at the ankle, and then hold it five seconds, followed by doing the same thing with your left arm and left leg. For further stretching of your legs and Achilles tendons, try straightening out your right leg with your right heel firmly on the floor, and then extending your left leg forward while slowly and slightly bending it at the knee and holding it in a flexed position for five seconds. Repeat this a few times, and then do the same with your left leg.

The range of quick and easy exercises and stretches that you can do in your office or workstation is as vast as you want to make it. More options comfortably include touching your toes, standing straight up and twisting your torso from one side to the other, shadowboxing, using your chair for balance exercises, forcefully pushing your hands together, locking your hands and then trying to pull them apart, extending your arms in front of you and moving them as if you're rowing a boat, extending your arms to the side and circling them clockwise and then counter-clockwise, and much more.

ACCESSORIZE AND EXERCISE

If you'd like to add more strengthening, calorie burning, and conditioning to the light exercises that you're doing while working at or around your desk, there are accessories just waiting to take you and your routines up a notch—and your weight down a notch. Some of them are probably on your desk right now, and they're free. If you have a stapler, a full water bottle, a paperweight, or any other decorative or functional item that weighs a pound or so, just pick it up and use it as a weight. Alternate from one arm to the other and do some curls, row a rowboat, flap like a bird, or reach for the sky. Also from the standpoint of using building supplies to build yourself up, how about placing a ream or two of paper on your lap as you sit, with the balls of your feet planted on the floor while you raise and lower your heels fifty times?

In addition to the freebies available within arm's reach, there are plenty of excellent light weights available in the marketplace today. In seeking out the right one for you, there's no need to go into bench press mode. Even something in the range of a pound or two can work very well. In fact, researchers at McMaster University in Ontario, Canada, found that more frequent lifting of lighter weight generates the same increases in muscle-building as lifting heavy weights. Plus, lighter weights work particularly well in your office, especially since they're likely to fit comfortably into your hands as well as into a briefcase, purse, or desk drawer.

In a Squeeze

Another way to introduce more activity and conditioning into your work is by using a couple of stress balls or squeeze balls. When you stand up to stretch or take a mini-stroll in your office or workstation, put one of these balls in each hand and squeeze. This helps strengthen your hands, fingers, forearms, and wrists, all the while burning a few extra calories. These balls can also come into play when a coworker comes into your office or workstation to pitch some ideas to you. Ask this person if she'd like to play some catch at the same time. Most will respond affirmatively. As your discussion continues, you're tossing the ball back and forth, and you're doing the same thing with ideas—bouncing them off each other. As you go through the physical actions of playing catch, you're engaging areas of your brain that typically don't come into play in a standard meeting or discussion. This can lead to innovative ways to approach lingering issues as well as insights that had been out of sight up to this point. Plus, as your pitch count goes up, so does the number of calories that you're expending.

Other accessories that can help you burn calories and build muscle tone in your office or workstation include hand grips, wrist weights, ankle weights, weighted belts, and weighted vests. If you put on these weights when you stand, stretch, or walk in your office or workstation, you're more likely to take off some weight as a result.

FURNITURE, FITNESS, AND FATNESS

By seizing every opportunity to work calories away, whether on your feet or in your seat, you're on your way to eliminating the key contributors to the sedentary nature of today's jobs and the weight gain that comes with it. While walking, stretching, and exercising will certainly help you win the battle of your bulge, you're likely to have a more resounding victory by enlisting some additional equipment on your side—all as part of your office or workstation.

Standing Desks and Risers

With so much research spelling out the widespread advantages of standing and disadvantages of sitting, particularly in relation to caloric expenditure and weight gain, it's nice to know there's a tool you can use to get your work done while simultaneously spending far more time on your feet. It's called a standing desk. These are adjustable desks that allow you to stand for as long as you want while carrying out your deskbound responsibilities, assignments, and tasks, all with your computer, monitor, and desktop items at the ideal level for you to stand and work. When you feel like sitting, just give the crank a few turns or the lever a squeeze to lower the desk, or push a button for an electric motor to do the same, and then you can quickly and easily go into temporary sitting mode. Whenever you're ready, you can raise the desk to a height that best fits your own height, allowing you to place your arms at ninety degree angles to the keyboard and make your stance comfortable and ergonomically sound. Many can be raised to fifty inches or more and lowered to thirty inches or less, and they're often available with side trays for storage, brackets for managing cables and cords, and a grounded power strip with power plugs and powered USB outlets.

At the same time, a cost-effective alternative to this free-standing standing desk is a desktop riser. It's typically an adjustable stand that sits on your current desk or a platform mounted on an adjustable arm. Either one allows you to easily raise and lower the height of your keyboard, monitor, and desktop stuff—essentially transforming your existing desk from a sitting desk to a standing desk, and then back again as you wish. In addition to the benefits associated with standing, early research is finding that standing desks are associated with increased productivity. It appears that you're more likely to be on your toes when you're standing.

Treadmill Desks

If you want to step things up a notch and engage in even more activity, conditioning, and weight loss while working at your desk, you just might be interested in a treadmill desk. True to its name, if you combine a standing desk with a treadmill, you get a tread-mill desk. Depending upon the make and model, treadmill desks can have features such as programs that count your steps, meas-ure your activity levels, and track your distance. Other options can include padded arm rests, sit-down and stand-up alerts, push-button height adjustments, and sufficient width for a chair when you want to lower the desk, do some sit-down work, and be totally off the treadmill—other than the figurative treadmill known as your job. If you already have a standing desk, it's not difficult to find a treadmill that fits perfectly underneath, known in the trade as an under desk treadmill. And if you already have a treadmill, there are standing desks that can fit over and around it as well. The idea behind all of these desks is that as you're work-ing, you're building your physical condition and burning calories by walking. And just to be clear, it's walking, not running. It's not a race or a chase, but just an easy pace. In fact, many of the tread-mills can be set to keep the pace at two miles per hour or less.

If these higher-energy desks sound tempting, here's one more point that might seal the deal. Researchers at the Mayo Clinic estimated that overweight office employees who replace sitting time on their computers with walking time on their computers by two to three hours each day could lose between forty-four and sixty-six pounds in the course of a year. To achieve these results, the pace doesn't have to be brisk—the users don't even need to break a sweat. Additionally, researchers at the Carlson School of Management at the University of Minnesota found that the adoption of treadmill workstations led to improvements in performance, work quality and quantity, and interaction with fellow employees. And further, the participants' overall physical activity levels per day also increased. By opting for these types of desks and sporting your pedometer all the while, the notion of 10,000 steps per day and the wellness and weight loss this can bring start to sound a lot more feasible and achievable.

Liking Biking

If you'd like to sit at your desk for long stretches on end, specifically on your end, there's a way to do so while still burning up calories and bringing down your weight. How can this be? Two words—bike desk. You can be pedaling away and gaining the benefits that come from biking and do so while working away at your desk. You actually have a wide variety of choices when considering bike desks. You can opt for a single unit that's essentially an exercise bike built into a standing desk or something as basic as an exercise bike with an attached desktop. Features can include adjustable seats and seat backs, storage compartments and drawers for your desktop items, adjustable arm rests, extra padding, ability to convert from upright to semi-recumbent, instruments to measure your progress, adjustable resistance, collapsibility for storing, and more.

Pedal Pushers

Let's say you prefer sitting at your standard desk and in your standard chair, but you'd be inclined to do some pedaling if the option were available. In fact, there are numerous under-the-desk pedal exercisers that you can slide right under your desk right now. Once it's in place, you can go ahead and sit in your standard chair and pedal to your heart's content. With a pedal height of approximately ten inches, these under-the-desk exercisers are lightweight, portable, and quite affordable, and they can come with any number of additional features that allow you to vary the resistance as well as measure your reps, speed, distance, time, calories burned, and more. All of these bike-like units can certainly put a dent in the sedentary nature of your job while helping you manage your weight and your work at the same time. They also give a new meaning to the term, business cycle.

Have a Ball

Another piece of office furniture that can help transport you from the sedentary era to the active era goes by several names—fitness ball, exercise ball, or stability ball. Sometimes it's simply a large ball that you roll up to your desk and use as a chair. Other models—ball chairs or balance ball chairs—use the same type of large ball mounted on frames that can include arm rests, casters, a back support, and several adjustable features. They come with a number of benefits and a number of issues. On the positive side, some experts contend that these chairs enhance muscle tone, improve posture, increase balance and stability, reduce back pain, and keep you moving while sitting. On the flipside, other experts aren't so supportive, especially in terms of the support these ball chairs provide. Such experts voice concern about the placement of extra pressure on your lower back, general discomfort, and even the possibility of the balls bursting. In other words, there are some experts who swear by these chairs and others who swear at them. Either way, the most common point of agreement is that sitting on these chairs causes calories to be burned. If these well-rounded seats are intriguing to you, the ball's in your court.

Get the Message

When making physical changes in your work area that can make physical changes in you, some experts extol the value of motivational messages. The idea is that these pithy phrases posted on your desktop, credenza, shelves, and other prominent points will provide you with ongoing reminders, support, and motivation to take actions to meet your weight loss goals. Just like advertising, when you see messages repeatedly over time, they start to sink in, gain an aura of truth and believability, and become part of your hardwiring. As a result, these messages can have a powerful impact on your behavior. Why not be your own ad agency and provide yourself with inspirational, motivational, and self-affirming messages that you can internalize and then actualize? They all have one shared objective—to encourage you to increase your activity level at work and thereby increase the likelihood of success in meeting your weight loss goals. In this regard, researchers found that the use of wrist-based or computerized prompts to remind people who are seated for an hour to stand up led to a reduction in average sitting time and an increase in average walking time, among other positive findings. In fact, the participants who were also prompted to walk at least one hundred steps experienced a significant increase in the number of steps per day at work. While posted reminders are transmitted differently from the prompts in this study, there's a direct parallel which can induce you to stand up and get moving. In terms of the exact phrasing, you can write your own messages or prompts to post around your work area such as, "I'm up for the challenge." "Reach for the stars. Take the stairs." "Walk for a change." "Take a stand." "Don't weight. Get up now." "Sitting is quitting." "I stand for health." "Don't sit around. Move around." "Get up. Get healthy." "Go out and stand. It's outstanding."

There's no question that today's jobs are more sedentary. But importantly, this doesn't mean that you have to be more sedentary.

Chapter 5

Let's Do Lunch

It used to be so easy. Like clockwork. The bell would ring, and you'd file out of your classroom for your designated lunch period. You'd take a break from the world of isosceles triangles, history, and biology quizzes so you could eat, chill out, chat with friends, and maybe run around the schoolyard. But much like your bygone school days, it's leisurely lunches that have actually gone bye-bye. Numerous jobs today are making it increasingly difficult to take a real lunch break, and workers are left in the lunch lurch. A study by Right Management found that just one in five workers takes an actual lunch break, with nearly a third of employees rarely taking a break, 14 percent who do so sporadically, and almost 40 percent who eat at their desks. Another survey by OfficeTeam found that approximately half of employees take thirty minutes or less for their lunch breaks, and almost a third of employees spend their lunch breaks working while eating. Why has the concept of a taking a real lunch break become so broken?

THE LUNCH CRUNCH

One prevalent feeling amongst working people is that there simply isn't enough time to carry out their daily responsibilities and still be able to leave their office or cube to sit down for a square meal. It seems impossible. As a result, employees wind up taking fast trips for fast food, eating fast while fastened to their desks, or even fasting throughout the entire day. The high demands placed upon employees, the lack of downtime, and the increased on-the-job pressures faced by millions each day are all contributing factors that are factoring out lunch. Proper lunch breaks take a backseat to projects, deadlines, reports, and presentations, and it's all too often that meetings that are planned to accommodate everyone's schedules are anything but accommodating to your lunch needs. And you're left shit out of luck and shit out of lunch.

Consumed by Technology

Technology also plays a key role in the vanishing lunch break since your phone, tablet, and computer keep you constantly connected to your work at all hours of the day. This can make taking a breather to physically and mentally separate yourself from work in order to eat far more challenging since you're always on call. Face it, when your boss dials you at noon, you're going to be picking up the phone instead of picking up your lunch order. Also, the globalization of the corporate world is yet another contributor to the diminishing lunch break, as different time zones may make your lunchtime the only time that you can connect with clients and associates in different regions and countries. So it's konnichiwa colleagues, sayonara lunch.

Job and Lunch Elimination

Additionally, you can blame the economy for taking a bite out of employee lunch breaks, since employees are now carrying even greater workloads due to employers who are cutting jobs and cutting costs. Employees fear that their jobs may be eliminated, and as departments get smaller and smaller, the need for employees to constantly prove themselves to their manager means that finishing a project takes precedence over finishing lunch. Some employees who take quick lunches, eat at their desks, or forgo lunch altogether also do so to show how busy, important, and critical they are to their department. Peer pressure from colleagues and managers is also preventing employees from utilizing their lunch breaks—they fear being viewed as slackers or as not having enough to do. Plus, forgoing lunch in some companies has come to mean that you're somehow more dedicated to your job than others. And if your employer is looking to promote an individual or eliminate a job, who appears more vital to the company—a person who works through lunch or a person who takes his full break? Suddenly you're on the chopping block because you left to take your lunch break around the block. In fact, there's a phrase that's heard in the background and foreground in many organizations today, "Lunch is for wimps."

TODAY'S LUNCHES

As real lunches and lunch breaks disappear across workplaces, more and more weight is appearing across the workforce. For an individual who manages to leave his workplace for lunch, there are potentially weighty pitfalls for those making a pit stop. Research has found that those who eat out for lunch generally consume around 158 extra calories during their meal. When looking at those calories in terms of a year, dining out for lunch adds an extra 39,500 calories, which is approximately eleven pounds, right off the bat. Plus, a study in the *Journal of the Acad-*

emy of Nutrition and Dietetics revealed that the eating habits of those with whom you dine can influence the amount that you eat. Namely, if you're going out to lunch with a bunch of suits from your office who order giant portions and tempting treats, you're more likely to follow suit. More shockingly, research has shown that diners who are simply informed that their peers are consuming high-caloric meals were still more likely to mimic this same detrimental dining behavior—even without actually seeing what their peers were eating. To that end, diners need to be wary of the built-in restaurant hazards such as tantalizing smells, sights, and sounds that fill the air and potentially their stomachs when dining out during the day. Eating out for lunch can be risky business for those in the business of losing weight.

In a Hurry

For employees who find themselves flying out of the office and downing whatever they can get their hands on, it should be noted that rushed eating can lead to weight gain. When you eat in a hurry, you can prevent your brain from having enough time to receive signals from your gut to determine that you're satiated, and therefore you're more likely to overeat. As noted by Harvard researchers, eating more slowly may help you feel fuller faster because you're giving your body the chance to recognize that you're full. As employees take shorter and shorter lunch breaks, they end up denying their bodies this important opportunity and often consume more than needed. Since the eateries frequently frequented by many fast-paced lunch-goers may contain fewer options when it comes to items that provide optimum health benefits, rushed eating is compounded by the types of foods that are getting overeaten. After all, when you're strapped for time and looking for a place that'll feed you in a flash, fast food restaurants tend to be the go-to stop. And yet constantly eating fast food, especially at a fast and furious pace, is only going to make you furious with yourself and your weight soon after.

Desk Diners

For those who are so busy that they eat their lunches at their desks, other fattening factors can come into play. If you find yourself eating lunch while working, you're likely to engage in distracted eating. It's this type of eating that can cause weight gain. After all, when you're concentrating on sending emails, analyzing data, and typing reports, it's difficult to concentrate on how much you're consuming. As a result, you're more likely to overeat. Preoccupied eating makes it more difficult to keep track of how hungry or full you are, and before you know it, you've read the email you wanted, but you've eaten far more than you wanted. Your inbox may no longer be full, but your stomach is. Desk-eaters are also denying their bodies and minds the opportunity to take a real break from their job, and research has consistently proven that without time to mentally and physically separate yourself from your work, you're more likely to experience lower levels of efficiency, creativity, and energy. Attempting to be productive during your lunch break can actually be counterproductive for you and your company.

Desk-dwellers also have some stickier issues to consider when lunching at their desks. Here's something to chew (or choke) on—how often do you clean your desk? If you turn over your keyboard, do crumbs fall out? A survey conducted by the American Dietetic Association and ConAgra Foods' Home Food Safety program revealed that only 36 percent of employees clean their work area during the workweek, and 64 percent of employees clean their work areas once a month or less. In fact, 30 percent of women and 45 percent of men reported that they seldom or never clean their work areas at all. Even more disturbing, a University of Arizona study revealed that desks have about one hundred times more bacteria than the average kitchen table and about 400 times more bacteria than the average toilet! That's right, you might as well be eating in an outhouse instead of in your office. And speaking of sickening, when you're distracted by work-related tasks while having lunch at your desk, it can be hard to keep track of how long your food has been sitting out. While you may think of yourself as a stellar employee who eats lunch while continuing to work, you're also exposing yourself to food-borne illness which can inevitably result in more sick days. In a word, eating at your desk may just put you hovering over a real toilet soon after.

Passing on Lunch

Then there are the lunch-skippers. Busy. Overworked. And under-fed. These individuals typically feel that because they're so pressed for time, their only options are to forgo eating lunch or even refrain from eating anything at all throughout the workday. But skipping meals only sets you up to stuff your face later. After all, humans are supposed to eat! And when the late afternoon rolls around and/or you come home from work famished, you often find yourself overeating because you're over-hungry. Not only is skipping meals associated with obesity, but as noted in the medical journal *Metabolism*, skipping meals during the day and then overeating at night causes dangerous metabolic changes such as higher fasting glucose levels and delayed insulin response which are conditions that can lead to type 2 diabetes. Additional concerns for lunch-skippers are the effects it has on their physical, mental, and cognitive state. As research has found, if you don't eat lunch while at work, you're likely to experience fatigue, tiredness, irritability, a lack of concentration, and poor decision-making—not the qualities you'd like to see on your performance appraisal.

For the meal skippers whose strategy is to grab a little something from whatever they can find around the office, these impromptu meals and faux-lunches aren't doing your body or your mind any favors. A study by CareerBuilder found that 8 percent of over 3,600 employees eat lunch from their companies' vending machines at least once a week. Of course, that's using the term "lunch" loosely, as opposed to the fit of their pants. Candy plus cookies plus chips doesn't equal lunch, as you're not giving your body what it really needs. You know this! When you skip meals, you're more likely to make crappy food choices and overeat the less-than-healthy and less-than-helpful items found in your workplace. If you had taken the time to plan ahead and have the right kinds of food available for yourself at work, the birthday brownies in the break room in honor of Anna from Accounting wouldn't seem so irresistible, and you wouldn't suddenly find yourself forcing them down in a famished and frantic state. Being levelheaded and keeping your hunger in check are essential components of weight control. Meal-skippers should also keep in mind that coffee isn't a meal replacement. Coffee in high doses is not only hazardous for your health, but solely consuming coffee is quite dangerous for a whole slew of reasons, including that it can lead to overeating. Your liquid lunch is actually a solid nightmare for your body.

REVIVING LUNCH

Incorporating a real lunch break that includes a healthy meal is an integral component for weight and work success. It's critical to find a midday stopping point that enables you to replenish, relax, and refocus. By redirecting your on-the-job and out-of-the-box (the lunch box) thinking toward your own lunch and lunch break, you'll enormously benefit work-wise, health-wise, and weight-wise without becoming enormous. Reality check—everyone's busy. Everyone's rushed. Everyone's got a million things to do. Get over it! When you're finished making excuses, you can start making changes. The good news is that there are several proven and palatable processes for you to employ so you can finally bring the power back to lunch.

In the Bag

How do you incorporate a real lunch into your corporate world? One key strategy is to brown bag it. Bringing your lunch to work is extremely beneficial as it enables you to completely control your lunch's food prep, contents, portion size, as well as cost. A common complaint from anti-brown-baggers is that there just isn't enough time to make a lunch. But a lack of time isn't an acceptable excuse in your work situation, so why should it be acceptable in this situation, especially when it comes to your health?

Manage your time just as you would for any other job-related assignment or task. Get up early. Pack your lunch the night before. Plan out your meals for the week. Do what you have to do to turn your lunch into a priority. It's not an option, but an obligation to put your health first. Plus, it's been shown that brown-bagging it can actually reduce your weekly lunch cost by 80 percent. Who couldn't use the extra money? Any savvy financial advisor and healthcare advisor would tell you to take advantage of bringing a lunch, as it's good for your wallet and your waistline. Additionally, brown-bagging it can prevent you from getting sucked in by all the tempting treats and fatty finds that you can't help but suck down when dining out for lunch. Brown bag lunches truly enable you to take charge of what you're consuming instead of the other way around.

Making Lunch Work for You

The trick to preparing a lunch for work is to use it as an opportunity to make the best food decisions for yourself and select items that'll help get you through the workday in every respect. Including lean protein into your lunch routine such as skinless white meat chicken, unprocessed turkey, salmon, eggs, and low-fat dairy can keep you fuller longer which helps to thwart overeating later in the day. Beans and lentils are also weight-friendly weapons to pack in your lunch arsenal as they're packed with protein and fiber which can help you stay full as well. Also, don't overlook fruits and vegetables. In fact, many of them are regarded as superfoods or brain foods that can help power you throughout the day without supersizing you.

Another go-to strategy for brown-baggers is to start off the week by purchasing salad ingredients such as lettuce, kale, or spinach leaves and produce such as tomatoes, bell peppers, beets, broccoli, cucumbers, carrots, and mushrooms, and then spice up your salad with special additions and fixings. That means one day's lunch can be a veggie-rich salad topped with an individual serving of tuna which is low in calories and high in protein and omega-3 fatty acids. Another day, you can spice up your salad with salsa, canned corn, low-fat cheese, avocado, and a serving of black beans. While your supermarket may also sell premade salads and salad kits with prewashed items that can save you time, beware that such salads may have more calories than you bargained for. Watch out for croutons, tortilla chips, and fattening dressings. Swap out these unhealthy items at home and add more of your favorite veggies as well as substitute the dressing with other selections you like—preferably an oil-based vinaigrette, as oils can help your body absorb key vitamins and nutrients. And don't be afraid to make your own salad dressing combination of olive oil and vinegar. It's a classic for a reason.

Sandwiched In

If your midday meal isn't complete without a sandwich or wrap, the first step is to select a whole grain bread or wrap and cover it with healthy items like onions, tomatoes, lettuce, spinach leaves, sprouts, and avocado. Try to include lean proteins like tuna and white meat chicken as well as low-fat cheeses, and don't forget that hardboiled eggs are also great sandwich and wrap stuffers. In terms of condiments, mustards, olive oil mayonnaise, hummus, and even mashed avocado can make great spreads. If you're worried that a soggy sandwich or wrap is going to put a damper on your lunch plans, you can always bring the ingredients packed separately and assemble the sandwich at work. Another option is to create a meat/cheese barrier against the bread or wrap and spread the condiments onto this layer while placing the wetter ingredients in between. Want another tip to help you get into tip-top shape? When preparing dinner for yourself, use your executive planning skills and make extra so that you can take some to work for lunch the next day. Before you even sit down for dinner, separate and pack up your lunch portion to save yourself time and eliminate the possibility of overeating at dinner.

Pack Smart

An additional element associated with bringing your lunch is not only what you pack, but how you pack. While the concept of brown-bagging your lunch is a work "do," an actual brown bag is a work "don't." Nearly half of American adults admit that they've left their lunches in need of refrigeration out for three hours or longer—the problem is that perishable items shouldn't be left out for more than two hours in order to prevent spoilage and food-related illnesses. When it comes to practicing safe lunch, invest in insulated lunch bags and ice packs, and don't forget to clean them. Put your lunch into the refrigerator or freezer immediately upon your arrival at work. Make it the first thing that you do when you get to the office, no matter how busy you are.

If your line of work prevents you from having access to a refrigerator and/or if no refrigerator is available at your workplace, don't let this spoil your brown-bagging plans or your lunch itself. Rather than relying on the unhealthy offerings of so many restaurants, if your job keeps you out of a physical workplace, purchase a cooler so that you can keep your lunch cold no matter where you are. Some oh-so-cool cooler tips are to store your cooler at home in a cool place so that it's not initially warm when packing it, fill it with icepacks, and place your foods into the cooler in the reverse order that you'll be accessing them during the day so as to prevent cold air from escaping every time you open and close the lid. To that end, you may even want to keep your beverages in a separate cooler if you're more likely to be opening and closing it more frequently through-out the workday. Another option is to fill your lunch with non-perishable food items that don't need refrigeration, such as peanut or almond butter sandwiches, fruits, vegetables, unopened precooked canned foods such as tuna, chicken, and salmon, and unopened packets of condiments.

Drink Up, Weight Down

When selecting a drink that'll accompany your lunch, whether you're dining at your office or out on the town, the best option is water. You know this. What you may not know is that water doesn't have to be boring, as it's actually an opportunity to get creative. There are many low-calorie water additions to choose from, such as a spritz of lime or lemon, sliced cucumber, a sprig of mint, frozen fruits like blueberries or strawberries, and even a splash of 100 percent fruit juice. There are also zero-calorie flavored waters that provide a tangy punch, and don't overlook unsweetened decaf iced tea. In fact, green tea is a superfood. The trick when selecting a beverage that works with your lunch is to not drink your calories. Respect your body, and put down the sugary sodas, milkshakes, and caloric-blended nightmares since they're only doing you harm. Water is known to help your kidneys, heart, bowels, skin, energy level, hydration, and even aid in keeping your weight down. And while water is not a magic treatment, other drink options are simply mistreating you.

UNLUCKY POTLUCK

A common practice in workplaces today is the potluck lunch. Employees decide whether as friends or as departments to bring dishes that'll each contribute to the greater meal for those involved. Potluckers usually decide ahead of time—or sometimes get assigned—certain components of the meal for which they're responsible such as appetizers, main courses, or desserts. In many instances, the specific contents of dishes that others are bringing aren't always known until lunch is served. While potlucks are a great way to boost camaraderie, cooperation, and morale, they can also boost your weight. Employees can easily fall victim to potential potluck potholes, such as overeating and peer pressure, as well as a general lack of food options that align with their weight goals. After all, the definition of the word "potluck" is a situation in which you're taking a chance that whatever's available is good or acceptable. But what happens when it's not?

The first step to turning a potluck in your favor is to be responsible for bringing an item that falls in line with your weight goals. That way, even if all of the other foods and dishes at the potluck range from unhealthy to unthinkable, you're guaranteed an option that's pleasing to your taste and your waist. It's up to you and you alone to make the best food choices for yourself, which is why you have to take charge and bring a healthy dish to the potluck. In terms of the actual dish or dishes you should dole out, the possibilities are endless as long as you do the grunt work. It's easy to bring fattening options such as potato chips and onion dip, cheesy casseroles, and fudge brownies, but it's anything but easy to burn off those calories later and turn off your feelings of remorse and regret. No matter what course of the meal you bring, the best course of action is to use your dish as an opportunity to put yourself at an advantage. Assigned an appetizer? Bring crudités with garlic hummus or salsa. Managing a main course? Bring a romaine salad with white meat chicken, feta cheese, tomato, olives, cucumber, and dressing on the side—for portion and sogginess control. Need a dessert? Supply your coworkers with your favorite fresh fruits and fat-free frozen yogurt.

Another potluck rule of thumb is the "one plate, one time" philosophy. That means use one plate and one plate only for your entire meal, and take only one trip through the potluck line. And that's it. With multiple plates and multiple visits, it's too hard to keep track of how much you're consuming, and this can inevitably lead to overeating. Also, be mindful of how much you're piling onto your plate as it's easy to take too much when so many different options are in front of you. Attending a potluck isn't an excuse to double or triple your lunch portion size unless you feel like striking out weight-wise. Slow down, take a deep breath, and go through the potluck line in control, selecting the foods that you want to eat and leaving behind the items that don't benefit your weight goals.

If peer pressure is alive and well in your organization, the first step is to be aware of it, and the next step is to deal with it. If you're getting sour treatment for not loading up on your co-worker's sweet treats, you have options to deal with this less-than-saccharine ridicule, just as you would deal with this same type of behavior in any work-related situation. First, you can always ignore it. Done and done. You can also defend or explain your actions, telling the ringleaders that you're full, not that hungry, don't feel like it, or that you may have one later—even if you don't intend to. The bottom line is that no one can make you eat something except for you. You're not pledging a frat! So stand up for yourself and your weight goals, and do what's right for you. If you want a cookie, have a cookie. If you don't, then don't. Just be sure that you're eating an item because you truly want it. If you know that you usually fall into the same old trap where one cookie leads to ten, don't sabotage yourself. Would you ever do that on a work project? Be honest with yourself, take responsibility, and put yourself in a position to succeed.

OUT TO LUNCH

If ordering food in or lunching out is either your choice or the choice of colleagues, clients, or customers, there are ways to make your working lunch work for you. If the restaurant is decided upon ahead of time, it's up to you to look at the menu and nutrition info online, get answers to how foods are prepared, read the reviews, look at dish photos, and do everything in your power to determine the most weight-and-waist-friendly option before you place your order or step into the restaurant. If a bunch of eateries are in contention, make sure you know what you'd possibly order at each of them. The information is there if you make the effort. You wouldn't approach any other work-related decision ill-prepared, so why do so here, especially when choosing what's going into your body? Even if the destinations are all fast food stops, and you feel caught between a rock and a fat place, you can still make the best meal choices for yourself given the circumstances by thoroughly preparing for whatever is being prepared for you. If you don't decide ahead of time, you risk ordering unhealthier items and perhaps succumbing to pressure from your coworkers in the heat of the moment. Additionally, a growing trend in restaurants today is to have a "guiltless section" or list of options that are below a certain number of calories that they proudly display on their physical and online menus. Knowledge is a powerful weight loss tool, so take advantage of the resources at your fingertips—whether online or on an app—which can help steer you in the right direction. By eradicating the guesswork and prospect of failure, just as you approach other serious work projects, you can pull off the working lunch and keep the weight off as well.

Local Flavor

Want another lunch tip? Use the location of your lunch as an opportunity to get some exercise. A great way to burn calories and give your mind and body a much-needed midday break is to literally and figuratively step away from your office and walk to where you'll be dining. Instead of dealing with packed streets and parking lots, pack some shoes (if need be) and arrive at your lunch destination via foot. Your new favorite restaurant might be just around the corner, so do the actual legwork and find out about the different food venues in your area. Plus, a major perk of dining at destinations in close proximity to your office is that many local eateries will often give coupons and discounts to employees of nearby companies in order to increase business. A short call to your HR manager can mean big dining savings for you and your colleagues. To this end, neighborhood restaurants may also be more inclined to prepare special orders and meals just for you. If you'd prefer a chicken breast grilled in olive oil instead of butter, a Cobb salad that swaps out bacon for more hardboiled egg, a sandwich without mayo but with extra mustard, or a side of fruit instead of a side roll, many local eateries will be more than happy to make accommodations in hopes of seeing you—and feeding you—again. And who knows, if you come back often enough, you may just end up with a dish named after you—a healthy dish.

WHAT THE TRUCK?

A relatively new lunch phenomenon today is the fleet of food trucks that has descended upon workplaces across the United States. These are not the trucks of old—or the old trucks—from days of yore, filled with premade sandwiches, candy bars, and other packaged snacks. Rather, today's trucks are now upscale, chic, trendy, and often referred to as "gourmet trucks," with many serving restaurant-quality dishes and offering menus as different as lions and lamb chops. In fact, these food trucks have become almost like celebrities, with social media followers galore and even food-truck-based reality shows.

On the one hand, food trucks and their accessibility to the working public are major pluses, since they provide you with an instant opportunity to find a truck in close proximity to your office, hopefully with fresh foods and healthy options that'll please your palate without pushing your pants size. In fact, there are apps that can help you easily locate and track the closest food trucks in your area, and the good news is that there are plenty of organic, vegetarian, and even vegan food trucks serving up delectable salads, quinoa bowls, and spinach wraps right from the farm. Food trucks also provide you with an opportunity and incentive to leave your workplace and take a calorie-burning stroll to and from the truck.

But there can also be a number of issues associated with these trucks, as it seems that many of them are simply fattening fast food eateries on wheels, offering tempting delights that are high in calories, carbs, and fat, such as a macaroni and cheese rib sandwich. While the picture of that sandwich may be worth a thousand words, it contains more than a thousand calories and will cause you to weigh more and feel a thousand times worse.

While there's certainly a novelty to these trucks, look both ways and proceed with caution, as many of these mobile eateries have nutritional information that may be difficult to locate online. However, since the cooks and chefs are usually highly accessible when ordering—in most cases right in front of you—inquire about how certain dishes can be altered for you so that they align with your weight loss goals. In many instances, you'll find that dedication to customers is more valuable than dedication to an exact recipe. Plus, if healthier items are what keep you returning for lunch day after day, it's in their best interest to serve you better. Having a sandwich wrapped in lettuce leaves, forgoing fatty sauces, and swapping out a side of fries for a side salad may be possible if you just ask.

LOCATION, LOCATION, LOCATION

Whether you're a brown-bagging diva or an ordering-in pro, when it's lunchtime at your office, don't eat at your desk. Instead, get up and go to the break room. Walk outside and find somewhere to enjoy your lunch, even if it means dining on steps or a staircase. You can always take your lunch with you and accompany your colleagues to the location where they're getting their food and sit with them at a community table. Do everything in your power to leave your desk so that you can have a moment to separate yourself from the grind. You might just find yourself collaborating with colleagues in new and different ways. Give your body and mind a much-needed midday break to unwind and refuel. This needs to be a priority each and every workday. Putting your phone away is also an important part of the process, even if it's just for a few minutes. Workplace psychologists agree that sitting at your desk all day is likely to interfere with your thinking and lessen your ability to work innovatively and creatively. If you want to improve your mental state as well as your weight, stepping away from your keyboard is key.

Doing the Noon-Walk

Speaking of stepping away, a great method to guarantee that you'll spend time away from your desk during lunch is to start a walking club. In many organizations, employees are coming together to take lunchtime strolls either before or after eating. It's abundantly clear that walking has numerous health benefits, including reducing the risk of coronary heart disease, certain types of cancers, and obesity, while also improving your blood sugar levels, blood pressure, as well as your mental well-being. Plus, you're burning calories.

Stuck to the Desk

Of course, there can be extenuating work circumstances that may prevent you from leaving your desk for lunch. Looming deadlines, last-minute projects, crises and firefights, emergency meetings, demanding clients, and workload overload, to name just a few. If you're in a position where you can't leave your desk for a lunch break, it's time to employ responsible eating. First, clean your desk both before and after eating, which means wiping down your keyboard, phone, and desktop, and even bringing a placemat. Your desk is not designed to double as a dining room table, so be sure to keep it sanitary. It's also important to bring the exact amount of food to your desk that you plan on eating for lunch, as it can be easy to overeat and difficult to keep track of portion sizes while sizing up your tasks. Just as you don't engage in distracted driving, don't engage in distracted eating. Plus, keep in mind the amount of time that your lunch has been sitting on your desk, since getting engrossed in work projects for long periods of time can cause gross things to happen to your food.

Most importantly, don't make a habit of desk dining. It's not healthy for you or your work. However, if you find yourself eating at your desk day after day, there may be larger issues that are actually causing you to become large. One of the central factors behind skipping lunch is time management. Take a look at the way you're prioritizing your work throughout the day and be willing to push lesser projects aside in order to handle the major ones. If you're encountering frequent interruptions that cause you to fall behind, deal with them in an assertive and business-like fashion and come back to them at a time that best suits you. Be willing to delegate and follow up. Plus, consistently monitor your time usage to be sure that you're making the best use of it throughout the day. By managing your time well, you can certainly manage to have a healthy lunch.

ALL WORK AND NO LUNCH

While stopping to eat a midday meal may seem impossible in many jobs, you're likely to be hungry throughout the day, scouring the halls in search of snacks, and stuffing your face later. Whether or not this lack of time for lunch is a regular occurrence or a once-in-a-while scenario, it's never been more crucial to have the appropriate foods with you to fuel you through your workday. Because guess what—even when you don't have time to eat, you still have time to eat. If you can make time for all of your other job commitments, you can make time to give your body what it really needs, as that's actually the most important commitment of all. To power and empower yourself on the job and keep weight gain at bay, another strategy for lunch skippers with seemingly no time to spare is to snack. And in order to control your snack options, bring them to work yourself. It's your responsibility. Don't rely on what may be lying around your office or hope that your daylong fast won't make you longing for cookies come four o'clock. You're just lying to yourself!

As a Matter of Snack

The good news is that there are plenty of hearty and healthy snacks that are full of nutrition, fiber, and protein that are no-muss and no-fuss for a fast-paced workday. Yogurt, string cheese, nuts, vegetables, and canned seafood and meat are great snack options to grab on the go when you don't have any downtime for a lunch time. Also, don't forget fruits like apples, blueberries, red grapes, strawberries, bananas, and cherries—all superfoods. You can easily transport them to work and have them available at your office so that they're ready for you when you're ready to eat. Plus, many of these items are available in prepackaged containers and forms which can make your life easier prep-wise, portion-control-wise, and clean-up-wise. That way, you won't have to take any spare time wondering how you're going to find something to eat at your workplace, and you won't have to rely on whatever's left over in the vending machine. You're not unprepared in work-mode, so don't be unprepared in weight-mode. Snacking on the right kinds of foods will provide you with the mental and physical energy you need to thrive throughout a demanding day, as a short-lived sugar rush is a waste for your waist.

When's the right time for snack time? Serious snackers look at their schedules as a whole and enter the times they're planning on snacking, even if it's only for a few minutes. Of course, schedules can change, and although there may be moments when things are up in the air, your daily work calendar can help eliminate some of the snacking guesswork, especially since you've already nailed down what your snack will be. At the same time, schedules can go both ways, and there may be days when meetings are rescheduled, conference calls are cancelled, and assignments are finished earlier than expected. The good news is that your snacks are always available to you when you need them. Whether you're planning to eat a yogurt between morning emails, a banana before the board meeting, and a can of tuna following the afternoon assignment, you have a predetermined schedule as a guide to help you through your busy day. Another added benefit is that when you consume these snacks at various points throughout the day, you're also keeping your blood sugar levels stable and managing your hunger. An orange is the new snack.

AS LUNCH WOULD HAVE IT

While incorporating a healthy lunch at work may take some work, many of today's most progressive companies are placing more importance on lunch, to the point that they're providing free and healthy lunches to their employees. These companies recognize that doing so generates competitive advantages that touch many key indicators of organizational effectiveness— employee wellness, productivity, motivation, morale, recruitment, and retention, along with upgrading a company's image and goodwill in all marketplaces. And further, when healthy food perks are available to employees, there's a greater opportunity for sharing ideas among colleagues since no one has to go "off campus" for lunch. This typically leads to increases in employee teamwork, communication, cooperation, coordination, and collaboration. Lunch is for wimps? Not even close.

Chapter 6

Prevent the Event
from Getting You

Along with a corporate landscape that's constantly glittered and littered with foodstuffs on which to stuff yourself, there's an entirely separate source of edibles that takes employees farther down the road to rotundity. This purveyor of portliness is none other than the plethora of celebratory events that crop up almost every day in organizations small and large—events that can easily take you from small to large. Regardless of whether these events are sponsored by the company or the employees, and regardless of the specific reasons behind them, the common denominator is that they involve eating, especially foods that are high in fat, calories, sugar, and carbohydrates. And one thing is certain—these events lead to weight gain. Eventually.

CONSUMPTION AT COMPANY EVENTS

It's not surprising that the prospect of partaking in company-sponsored events is greeted with open arms and mouths. In addition to hanging out with friends and teammates, plus getting a break from work, there's a deeper reason why employee attraction to these events is so compelling. It's part of your early hardwiring. You grew up linking food with any number of positive special occasions, to the point that eating and celebrating are inexorably intertwined today. If you think of an event, you're likely to think of a special food associated with it.

To show you just how powerful this relationship is, try a simple word association exercise. Think of a holiday and the first words that you associate with it. By doing so, you're likely to respond with foods that match the festivity. Halloween? Candy. Thanksgiving? Pumpkin pie. What about winter holidays, such as Christmas, Hanukkah, or Kwanzaa? A feast. In fact, if you look up the word "holiday" in a thesaurus, one of the synonyms is "feast." Is it any wonder why events and foods are so tightly interwoven in your mental programming?

Hippy Holidays

When companies hold special events to commemorate holidays, it's only natural for employees to drop their defenses and pick up the knife, fork, spoon, and calories. Beyond the hardwiring factor, when it comes to holiday celebrations at work, employees traditionally expect their company to offer traditional foods. For the employer, breaking traditions associated with holiday foods is an easy way to break morale and motivation. As a result, whether it's Presidents Day or Labor Day (or Bastille Day), the overarching attitude of employers is "let them eat cake." And the overarching attitude of the employees is to do so.

The idea of upholding traditions and meeting employee expectations plays a central role in determining the offerings at these events. Employees have come to expect candy on Halloween, lest they feel tricked. And management doesn't want to be that stodgy neighbor who turns out all of the lights on Halloween, so they let the candy flow. This also means green goodies on St. Paddy's Day, chocolate sweets on Valentine's Day, and a horn of plenty of calories around the winter holidays. If a company is closed on a major holiday, there often is some sort of an eating event before the closure with foods that closely comply with the traditional fare for that holiday. If the company is open on the holiday, the food fest often occurs on the holiday itself. Unfortunately, regardless of the timing of the celebration, the offerings are typically nothing to celebrate. But what would these events be without these foods? Probably a lot healthier.

Take a look at a typical menu for an employer-sponsored winter holiday luncheon at work. It's likely to include a potpourri of such items as Caesar salad, rolls with butter, macaroni and cheese, mashed potatoes with gravy, glazed turkey, glazed ham, sautéed carrots, plus an assortment of pies, brownies, and cookies. While it would be healthier to take a holiday from these kinds of company events, they're just the tip of the ice cream.

Pouring Food into Feedback

Employers frequently use food as a key component in individual, departmental, and companywide recognition programs. As a result, when recognition is focused on one employee, such as for his suggestions for improvements in the workplace, the reward is likely to be some form of caloric congratulations. One popular offering is a gift card to a local fast food eatery, but in some scenarios, perhaps fasting would make more sense than fast food. When the recognition is to commemorate a department's achievements, it's another food fest, commonly a meal, whether onsite or off. In either case, rather than focusing on the smorgasbord of compelling non-ingestible incentives, managers easily fall into the food/feedback trap, eliminating non-food rewards and focusing attention on food-oriented recognition.

On a broader scale, when there are companywide accomplishments, there's likely to be a large-scale congratulatory event of one sort or another. If the accomplishment is particularly groundbreaking, the reward can easily be another feast. And if it's not a sit-down meal ordeal, management typically sends out an email announcing that certain goals have been surpassed, adding that all of the employees deserve the credit for the outstanding results. The email goes on to say that everyone will be given a special treat to commemorate the landmark. That treat is a codeword for calories, carbs, fat, and sugar. Some of the more common offerings in this scenario include cupcakes, candies, mini-cakes, kettle corn, and ice cream. If you like flowcharts, the formula is that increased sales yield increased revenues which yield increased pounds—and not pounds sterling.

If you step back a bit, you'll see that this situation sounds a lot like an old psychology experiment on classic conditioning. The subjects of the experiment—the humans—engage in a positive behavior, and this is followed by a tasty pellet. Every time the humans engage in a behavior that the experimenter—the employer—wants them to repeat, a treat, snack, or feast is provided. As a result, the humans continue their positive behaviors in pursuit of these rewards, and the employer continues providing the pellets when merited by human behavior. However, when the subjects of the experiment step on the scale, they're likely to find that these rewards are not so rewarding. This is not to denigrate the motivations, thoughtfulness, or kindness of management in these instances. Management means well, but the employees swell.

Just Because

Speaking of managerial kindness, there are other times when employers want to give employees a treat simply as a way of letting them know they're valued and appreciated. These events are not intended to commemorate anything, but rather are intended to send a positive message to the team and give morale a boost. In most cases, these offerings also boost the employees' intake of fat, sugar, and calories, which again leads to a boost in poundage. This uptick occurs because the acts of goodness cover a vast array of diet busters, such as platters of bagels and cream cheese, endless trays of cookies, burgers, grilled cheese sandwiches, esoteric foods, all varieties of ice creams and pastries, and chocolate fountains.

As a side note, some members of management push even harder for these events because they create an opportunity for direct contact with the employees in a positive context. While savoring a sweet treat, employees tend be more positively predisposed in their interaction with management. It's tough to be tough when holding a brownie in one hand and a chocolate chip cookie in the other. After all, if management were to call a meeting to discuss any number of corporate changes, developments, or issues with large numbers of employees and do so without any edible offerings, many employees would stay away or attend in a distasteful state of mind. It turns out that the food served at these events actually serves as both an incentive and icebreaker.

EATEN UP AT EMPLOYEE EVENTS

There are special days in your life, both on and off the job, that your coworkers are likely to identify as occasions to celebrate.

Your birthday, anniversary with the company, engagement, forthcoming wedding, baby shower, birth of your child, wedding anniversary, promotion, and a new title all fall into this category, along with any number of additional individual milestones that you may have reached. When these blips hit your coworkers' radar screens, it's not long before an event is in the works.

In the planning stage for these types of events, one of the most important considerations is the food. What should it be? Who's going to bring it? How much is needed? In many cases, there's a turf war over who gets to bring in the goodies, and as a sign of true organizational teamwork and collaboration, your coworkers agree that anyone and everyone can bring in anything. It's more food, and that means more fun—and more fat.

But don't think you're too special, since this scene is replayed for every employee in your department and the landmarks in their lives. Do the math. Assume you have ten coworkers in your department, and each has two such events per year. That's another twenty days with additional cake, cookies, brownies, ice cream, and the like, all on top of the corporate foodscape and company-sponsored events. In addition, surely you have friends in other departments, and they have their own special events and the same ordeals. When cake and other sugary offerings are served in these departments at your friends' events, your friends probably want you to participate in the celebration as well. Perhaps you go to the event, and if you do, the first instruction you'll probably receive is to eat. And if you're busy and unable to attend? No problem! Your friends are likely to go wide with these events, and if you can't join in, they'll simply have a slice of cake dropped off at your desk. Just keep in mind that when your friends go wide, you get wide.

Celebrating Non-Events

Beyond the eating events associated with actual milestones in your life and the lives of your coworkers, there's an assortment of employee-sponsored events for incidents that don't truly merit much in the way of celebration, particularly in the workplace. Nonetheless, cadres of coworkers inflate these incidents into landmarks, and then gleefully orchestrate and celebrate events around them. It's the food fest for the employee who's about to go on vacation or has just returned from one, the bash for the coworker who's changing apartments, or the goodbye and good luck event for a colleague who's about to have a bunion removed. As for orchestrating such events, there are even made-up songs that go along with some of them. Do these incidents really merit a full-blown event? Hardly. It's very sweet of coworkers to put all of this together, but in reality, it's too sweet.

There are lesser-known holidays that typically remain in the background, unless event-hungry employees dig them out and make them the basis for even more food fests. With a little looking, it's not difficult to find holidays for almost every day of the year. Granted that many of them score high on the obscure scale, that fact can make them even more enticing for employees who thrive on celebrations. Perhaps some of your coworkers have already spotted and orchestrated events for such holidays as National Pie Day (January 23rd), Chocolate Mint Day (February 19th), International No Diet Day (May 6th), National Fudge Day (June 16th), National Cheesecake Day (July 30th), National Ice Cream Cone Day (September 22nd), and National Cake Day (November 26th). For your fellow employees who prowl for reasons to put on yet another carbs-and-cals event, the possibilities are a click away.

Then there are the employee-sponsored events that set aside all pretenses of celebrating achievements, accomplishments, or milestones, and directly focus on celebrating food and nothing else. One of the more common entrants in this category is the bake off. The idea is for employees within or between departments to bake something at home, bring it into work for an eating test and fest, and then have a vote to determine the winner. If it's a matter of which food tastes the best, the winner is very likely to be the offering that contains the most butter, sugar, and fat. This whole activity is yet another compelling opportunity for employees to consume unhealthy foods, all as part of a fun activity that includes cheers and jeers with your peers. Before you know it, you've sampled everything, and you have no idea of the amount of fattening ingredients that you just ingested. But your scale will provide the answer.

IMMEDIATE STEPS TO MEDIATE THE DAMAGE

If you'd like to keep the weight gain associated with company and employee events at a minimum, there are some strategies you can implement right now to help you meet this goal. First, as in all other areas of controlling weight gain on the job, you need a plan to deal with these events. When you walk into that break room or conference room filled with festivity and dietary temptations, you should already have a strategy locked securely in your mind, plus a commitment to stick with it.

Prior to the bash, you should contact whoever's throwing it and find out what's being served. If there are items that are in sync with your weight loss goals and strategies, make a mental note of them and befriend them when you arrive. If the entire menu spells dietary disaster, plan on going into prevent defense at this event. This mode means that you decide in advance to eliminate the options that are disruptive to your plan, take small portions of those that pose the least destructive elements, and remember that you don't have to lick the plate clean. A few bites will more than suffice. Keep in mind that much of this is occurring at work and during work hours. Presumably, you have other responsibilities and commitments, so don't feel that you have to attend every event, lest you'll find yourself diving into foods on National Learn to Swim Day (May 17th).

You may find it easier to stick with your plan if you have a teammate with you. If you have a fellow employee who's also trying to avoid the inflationary impact of these types of events, plan on attending with her and sticking together at the gathering. It's often easier for two committed people to maintain dietary restraint than it is for one. With a buddy at your side, you're less likely to get sidetracked.

Desk Drop-offs

How many times have you returned to your desk and found a piece of cake just sitting there, a plastic fork standing at attention in the middle? There's no note explaining its presence. If you're like most employees, you ate the cake. You probably assumed that it came from a coworker, and you reasoned that you'll find out the specific who's, what's, and why's soon enough. It's really a matter of eating now and asking questions later. But really, if an assignment appeared on your desk with no explanation whatsoever, would you immerse yourself in it? Slim chance. Why not apply the same thinking when it comes to foods that appear on your desk? You weren't thinking about cake, you didn't know it existed until five seconds ago, and you don't need it.

Bakeoff Backfires

Then there are the tempting mysterious morsels that are served up at bakeoffs. With no information on the ingredients, you can easily end up partaking when you should be forsaking. These dishes may look inviting, but the odds are that they contain a mixture of many ingredients that can turn your plan into flan. It'll make more sense to flip into job mode and ask yourself how you'd handle a work situation that paralleled a bakeoff. With this in mind, if you received an email with a tempting offer for you to download, but you didn't know what it contained or what it would do to your system, would you do it? Of course not. Then why are you willing to download foods into your body's system without knowing what they contain? If this is how bakeoffs occur in your company, here's a simple piece of advice—when you hear there's a bakeoff, back off. At the same time, if you feel you must attend, it's okay for you to do some tasting, but the decision to eat anything is up to you—not your peers.

MIDTERM STEPS TO MITIGATE THE DAMAGE

Beyond creating, implementing, and following your own plan when attending these events, your next step is to do all in your power to generate some enlightened thinking regarding the foods that are offered at these events in the first place. This is relatively easy when it comes to events that are orchestrated by your fellow employees, since you can meet with them and openly share your ideas and suggestions, as well as show them tasty and healthy foods by bringing some to these events. This doesn't mean that you should show up with a bushel of broccoli for a coworker's birthday, but you can hit the health food section and bakeries in many markets and find healthier cakes, cookies, and sweet treats. Further, if you want to demonstrate your baking prowess, recipes for healthier sweets abound on the Internet. This can easily lead to cakes, cupcakes, cookies, and brownies that you and your coworkers will celebrate in every respect. There's also the option of deleting the bakery items altogether and celebrating these events with nuts and fresh and dried fruits. This could be the start of something big. And small.

The concept of healthier events also applies to employee bake-offs. However, just for the health of it, there are a couple of new guidelines to add. First, all of the items that are prepared for these contests will need to use healthy ingredients, and secondly, all of the ingredients have to be spelled out. As in so many aspects of work, competition is motivational, and by having employees compete in preparing the tastiest and healthiest foods, many new ideas about eating will be brought to the fore for the bakers as well as the biters. And the fun, excitement, enthusiasm, and pride associated with these bakeoffs will continue to heat up.

In Good Company

The process is a little different for company-sponsored events. If you're in a managerial position, you can use some of the power and influence inherent in your role to make some healthy suggestions for these events. If you're not in management yet, you still can play a key role in introducing this type of change in your organization, depending on the culture. If your workplace includes a warm, friendly, and supportive atmosphere in which employees' ideas and input are sought and acted upon, you should step up and make suggestions in this arena. However, if your company's culture is more influenced by past practices than forward thinking, and if the lines of communication tend to be primarily top-to-bottom, one way that you can still make your voice heard is to team up with like-minded coworkers and present your thoughts and ideas about healthier eating to management. Regardless of your job level and the approach that you use, make sure that management understands the potential benefits associated with your suggestions in this area, such as increased productivity, reduced absenteeism, increased energy, and possibly lower insurance costs. At the very least, suggest that management go with healthy offerings as a one-time trial for the next event. When it comes to changing individual behavior and organizational practices, it's much easier to take the plunge by starting on a trial basis. After all, most people are very reluctant to say, "No, I won't even give it a try." If the trial receives rave reviews, the following event is highly likely to incorporate healthy offerings, too. And so would the events that follow it. In light of this potentially widespread positive impact, if management agrees to go with a trial basis, you should try to involve yourself in the process to make sure that the healthier approach is given a healthy shot.

The introduction of healthier foods into the events at your workplace should touch every gathering in which employees touch food. Holidays. Obscure holidays. Recognition events. Employee milestones. General thank-yous. They're all food events, and they should provide goodies that do good and offerings that contribute to the employee's worth rather than girth. Take the winter holiday luncheon. Looking back at the typical menu noted earlier, a few replacements can easily turn a heavy table into a healthier tableau, thereby keeping cellulite out of the celebration. The first move is to remove the Caesar dressing from the salad and replace it with a low-cal balsamic dressing or simple oil and vinegar. As for the rolls with butter, drop in whole grain rolls and switch the butter for a healthier alternative such as a trans-fat-free buttery spread. If you absolutely must have pasta, consider whole grain noodles, tomato-based sauce, and Parmesan cheese. Mashed potatoes and gravy? Try baked yams. Glazed turkey and glazed ham? Have them deglazed. And the sautéed carrots? Say au revoir to the sauté and go with steamed. What about the assortment of pies, brownies, and cookies? Trade them in for fresh fruit with nonfat whipped topping as well as sugar-free cookies. With these substitutions, the meal still contains the flair of traditional fare, while the variety and flavor will surely keep the spirit bright.

Lightening the Load at Lunch-and-Learns

This strategy also applies to the increasingly popular lunch-and-learn sessions that are designed to provide employees with up-to-date information on issues, changes, and developments that are important to their work, personal development, and job performance, all in a comfortable and relaxed setting. As their name implies, lunch is served, and that can be a problem. While it's quite positive that these sessions contribute to employee growth, the food that's provided can cause the employees to grow in a different way, and that's not so positive.

When it comes to food at lunch-and-learn sessions, it's not uncommon to find such fat enhancers as pizza, processed sodium-laden sandwiches, potato chips, potato salad, and soft drinks, all followed by cookies and cake. No matter how you slice it, these sessions end up being a one hour sit-a-thon in which the attendees are likely to absorb a lot more than knowledge. Fortunately, this is yet another company event in which it's easy to eliminate the traditionally unhealthy offerings and replace them with foods that are just as tasty, but with far less fat, sugar, calories, and carbs. As one alternative, some companies are going Mediterranean for lunch-and-learns, and this means grilled or broiled chicken and fish, whole grain breads, olive oil instead of butter, fruits and vegetables, salads, nuts, and dairy products such as low-fat cheeses and yogurt. Not only do the attendees have a delicious and healthy meal, but there's a more subtle factor at work as well. When employees attend a lunch-and-learn, they typically come in with an expectation that they're going to learn something. By having this mindset, they're indeed more likely to learn—not only in terms of the material at hand, but also beyond the planned topics. As they focus on the information being presented, many of them are enjoying the healthy meal, and this is a learning experience as well. In fact, it's called experiential learning. By the end of the session, the attendees are likely to have learned something about the material that was presented, as well as something about themselves and the reality of eating healthy foods. For a double impact, just think how this plays out when the topic of the lunch-and-learn is "Healthy Eating at Work."

As a side note, research has found that a Mediterranean diet not only helps you control your weight and waist, it just might help lengthen your life. In a study of 4,600 women conducted at Brigham and Women's Hospital in Boston, participants who followed a Mediterranean diet had longer telomeres—the aging markers at the end of every chromosome in the human body. Longer telomeres are indicators of a longer lifespan, while shorter telomeres are linked to age-related diseases and a shorter lifespan. In addition, many studies have found that this diet also reduces the risk of heart disease, cancer, type 2 diabetes, stroke, and memory loss. Clearly, it's a memorable diet.

LONGER-TERM STEPS TO MITIGATE THE DAMAGE

Looking farther down the road, the goal is to break the food chain that links company events to eating. On the one hand, this isn't to say that all company events must be food free. It's entirely appropriate to have food—especially foods that aren't diet busters—at some events, such as a winter holiday luncheon or a birthday celebration. However, there's no need for food to be an inherent part of the huge number of other events where it now makes a center-stage appearance. If you really want to get a handle on preventing your job from giving you handles, the habit of automatically including food at company events needs to be broken.

Once again, if you're in management, you can manage to make this happen by using the same strategies and techniques previously mentioned regarding the introduction of healthier foods to these events. And if you're on the path to management, the same teamwork approach that was noted earlier is the way to go. However, as you make your case, be sure to do more than merely express concern or dissatisfaction regarding the extent to which present events are eating events. Instead, just as you'd deal with any other situation that poses risks, costs, and damages to the employees and company at large, you should come in with suggestions, strategies, and solutions.

Off the Recognition Chuck Wagon

One of the first steps is to realize that recognition doesn't have to come in the form of food. Using meals, treats, or food-based gift cards to recognize employee accomplishments and milestones is actually a very limited way to provide employees with reinforcement. To be truly meaningful, motivational, and satisfying, recognition should be tailored to the individual recipient, rather than a generic food offering that goes to everyone and anyone for just about anything. Many employees regard such offerings as little more than a perfunctory gesture. And worse, not only are far too many of these edible rewards laden with fat, carbs, and sugar, the recipients feel obligated to partake, lest they insult the hand that feeds them.

Rather than rewarding employees with free food, there are many food-free ways to provide recognition that are far more healthy, motivational, memorable, and personally significant for the recipients. With food-free recognition that truly fits the employee and his achievements and milestones, there's a long-lasting positive impact. With food-filled recognition, there's also a long-lasting impact, but it's usually found around the hips, waist, and thighs.

As food is removed from the recognition menu, there remains a vast array of methods to provide the employees with reinforcement that truly means something to them, moves them, and motivates them. Just to give you a taste, some of these techniques include a spot bonus, an afternoon off with pay, being featured on the company's homepage or website, a plant for the employee's office or workstation, a complimentary massage, a piece of art, an engraved plaque or trophy, placing the employee's name on a company Wall of Fame, a piece of inscribed jewelry, a personalized congratulatory card, a donation to a charity that's important to the employee, handwritten notes, paid trips, and free tickets to sporting events, plays, and movies. The list goes on, but the pounds don't.

By providing recognition without the seemingly requisite food offerings, the first link that binds eating to events is broken. This sets the stage for the introduction of additional company events that are totally free of food. However, the objective isn't simply to have food-free events, but rather to have outstanding events that stand out on their own while simultaneously doing wonders for employee morale, motivation, camaraderie, enjoyment, and satisfaction. Instead of having events contribute to employee weight gain, how about events that contribute to employee gains in knowledge, energy, strength, flexibility, self-esteem, self-confidence, and health? Now that's something to chew on.

Walk the Walk

When it comes to popular events that are having a major run in a growing number of companies, one of the top contenders is a walking program. By design, a walking program is structured to encourage, enable, and incentivize employees to combat the problems of long-term sitting and engage in one of the healthiest behaviors of all, walking. In these programs, interested employees sign up and receive guidance, support, and encouragement to make time to do more walking. In order to keep things interesting and fun, there's often a competitive element, with participants competing against themselves and against others, not only one-on-one but on teams as well, all in an effort to see who has walked the most steps in given time periods.

The incentives generally start early, often with a gift for signing up, be it a hat, shirt, or water bottle. Also from the get-go, one of the first and most important items is a pedometer. This is a handy device that, as its name implies, measures every step you take. In some programs, you'd buy the pedometer, while in others it would be supplied by your company, insurance agents, or an outside firm that specializes in "running" these programs.

Most pedometers clip onto a waistband or belt, while some are available as bracelets and others can be placed in a pocket, purse, or briefcase. If you're the buyer, the price can range from a few dollars all the way to hundreds. The features range from simply measuring the number of steps that you take and possibly converting them to miles or kilometers, all the way syncing with your computer and providing a vast array of data—your heart rate at various points along your walk, detailed tracking of your progress, analyses of how you slept, the number of flights of stairs that you've climbed, updated standings vis-à-vis the competition, and more. Whether you choose an app, a clip-on device, or even a smartwatch, any of them will help you move toward your walking goals.

Whether your company has designated a person to run the program, or if it's retained an outside firm to do so, the more common practices include initial benchmarking and tracking the number of steps that the participating employees take each week, plus ongoing feedback, encouragement, and advice along the way, often via social media. These communications also include information regarding the employees who have taken the most steps, as well as those who have met or exceeded their goals. At various points, there are prizes and incentives, such as headsets, running shoes, gift cards, and discount cards. At the end of the event, typically eight to ten weeks, each participant's mileage is totaled up, and the individual and group winners are announced. At that time, there are grand prizes that can include cash, tablets, laptops, and more. There's also a good deal of formal recognition through announcements and postings, along with more traditional recognition such as trophies and plaques. If an employee has physical limitations that prevent her from participating in these programs, most offer tailor-made wellness alternatives that suit the employee's condition and offer similar prizes.

Many of these walking programs establish a daily goal of 10,000 steps, a number that has been bandied about for years and is frequently cited as the baseline objective in various studies and by fitness experts. At the same time, this number is not cast in stone. The Centers for Disease Control and Prevention recommends that adults engage in 150 minutes of moderate level activity each week, with one such activity being brisk walking. Translating this into daily steps, wellness and exercise researchers indicate you'd need to walk in the neighborhood of 7,000 to 8,000 steps each day. The bottom line is that the baseline numbers and goals are best tailored to you and your company's program. Regardless of the benchmark number, with all of the promotion, plus online and offline chatter, these programs generate high levels of fun, teamwork, spirited competition, excitement, enthusiasm, and heightened interest in personal wellness and fitness.

If you step back and look at walking programs, it's not surprising that studies continue to find that they're correlated with weight loss. After all, if you're walking around rather than sitting around, you're burning calories. However, there's a more subtle element that compounds the power and effectiveness of walking programs, and it's all related to pedometers. In a study conducted at Stanford University School of Medicine, it was found that simply wearing a pedometer is linked to increased physical activity and weight loss. Further, it was determined that wearing a pedometer is associated with an increase of more than 2,000 steps per day which is approximately one additional mile walked each day. Plus, when it comes to walking programs, the researchers found that having specific goals regarding the number of steps to be taken per day was linked to greater levels of physical activity. Thus, while walking programs and their pedometers, awards, incentives, competition, camaraderie, and individual goals certainly spur the participants to use their feet more often, the mere act of wearing a pedometer is a major inducement to additional walking in and of itself. Apparently, simply knowing that you've got your pedometer clipped to you is enough to cause you to take some steps rather than take it easy.

A Fair Alternative

How about an event that by its very name discourages unhealthy eating? It's a health fair. The idea behind these fairs is to set aside a block of time, often two to four hours, along with a block of space, such as in your company's break room, parking lot, or a nearby facility, and invite the employees to come and meet with representatives from a broad array of health-related organizations. With a large number of welcoming booths that represent myriad wellness entities, these fairs provide your employees with a firsthand opportunity to quickly, easily, and comfortably engage in all sorts of interactions that are specifically designed to increase their knowledge and improve their health.

The mixture of exhibitors at these fairs covers the healthcare gamut, meaning that the presenters can check you out from head to toe. There can be presenters who provide vision and glaucoma tests, BMI screenings, blood pressure testing, bone health reviews, dental screenings, exercise and fitness advice, strength assessments, nutritional advice, skin care evaluations, massages, blood sugar testing, cholesterol screenings, breast cancer screening information, foot evaluations, and much more. In fact, these fairs can have as many presenters as the employees would like, as the health-related services that are represented can be directly tailored to the needs and interests of the employees.

With a little outreach into the medical community, it's not difficult for employers to organize these fairs on their own. At the same time, there are organizations that'll do all of the planning, organizing, and implementing of these fairs for your company—free of charge. A quick online search regarding these fairs will easily point you in the right direction.

A less obvious advantage of these fairs is that employees walk around from booth to booth, and this means extra steps if they're in the walking program. By attending the fair, they hit the trifecta—they're getting exercise by walking, they're getting professional advice and making contacts that'll improve their wellness and well-being, and they're getting a few steps closer to winning the prize in the walking program. That's more than a fair outcome.

Go with Yoga

Corporate yoga is another popular food-free program—it's a bit of a stretch, but in a good way. In these sessions, highly skilled yoga teachers come to the workplace and provide yoga training to all interested employees. The classes can be conducted before work, during lunch, and after work as well, and any size group can attend. Corporate yoga sessions typically include a combination of easy and gentle stretching, breathing exercises, and concentration techniques. The documented benefits of yoga reach into many areas, including increased strength, flexibility, bone health, muscle relief, muscle tone, relaxation, focus, mindfulness, self-insight, and concentration, along with reductions in tension, stress, and fatigue. As side benefits, these programs have been found to increase employee teamwork, cooperation, camaraderie, spirit, satisfaction, and morale. Additionally, researchers at the University of Oslo found that the practice of yoga can have a rapid, major, and positive impact on gene expression, especially in immune cells. In terms of the workplace, this means that yoga's direct contribution to immune system enhancement further increases the likelihood that yoga will lead to reduced levels of absenteeism.

Losers Who Win

One of the most powerful and popular events at work is a weight loss competition. It can be sponsored by the employees or the employer, and it's surprisingly easy to introduce and operate. If it's employee-sponsored, you or one of your buddies can simply announce that you're having this contest for whoever is interested. The participants would contribute a small agreed-upon amount, and they can participate as individuals or on teams. The prizes would come from the cash that's collected. If it's employer-sponsored, one point-person would oversee the program, and the prizes can be cash, merchandise, trophies, or even extra time off. These contests tend to run from four to twelve weeks, and that determination is totally up to the participants. There are also websites specifically designed to coordinate weight loss competitions. They help set up weight loss challenges, track individual and team weight loss with graphs and leader boards, provide interesting articles and fun facts, transmit upbeat and amusing weight loss banter, keep the levels of enthusiasm and competition high, and monitor which individuals and teams are losing and thereby winning. With all of the interaction, collaboration, and spirited competition, these programs introduce high levels of fun, interest, enthusiasm, and camaraderie into the weight loss process.

As for the effectiveness of these programs, there is considerable evidence indicating that competitive weight loss programs at work truly work. And things get even better when a little money is on the table. In a study of employees at Children's Hospital of Pennsylvania, one central finding was that attaching money to weight loss generated positive results, but the combination of money plus competition led to even greater weight loss outcomes.

Even More Events

It's as easy as pie to introduce employee-sponsored and company-sponsored events that are free of food yet filled with fun. Large numbers of popular events populate the food-free category, such as discounted gym memberships, a cookbook filled with the employees' healthiest recipes, incentives for walking or riding a bike to work, company sports teams, professional massages, outside expert speakers, community walks, volunteering and social outreach, and sponsoring and coaching youth sports teams. By the way, if you're looking for more food-free fun events that the employees will enjoy, some of the best ideas will come from the employees themselves. As is the case regarding the introduction of change in virtually any aspect of work, the more opportunities that employees have to provide ideas and inputs, the better the quality of the change and the more committed the employees will be to whatever's introduced. And this certainly applies to food-free events.

Chapter 7

Shedding the Heavy Burden of Job Stress

It's abundantly evident that the workplace is fertile ground for employee weight gain. However, there's a sinister underlying factor that exponentially increases the likelihood that today's workers are destined to put on extra pounds—stress.

Numerous studies show that workplace stress has been continuing to increase over the years. In fact, in the 2013 Work Stress Survey conducted by Harris Interactive, one central finding was that more than eight in ten employees in the United States indicated that they're "stressed out" on their jobs. Along these lines, the American Institute of Stress has determined that job stress is the greatest source of stress for adults in the United States.

With job stress at crescendo, the next piece is the inexorable link between job stress and gaining weight. When employees are asked how they handle the constant onslaught of stress on the job, some take the cathartic approach and say, "I scream!" while a far greater percentage take the caloric approach and say, "Ice cream!" The reason is that job stress and unhealthy eating are joined at the hip—or more accurately, the hips. This connection has been confirmed in numerous studies, including a major research project conducted through the University of Rochester Medical Center which further demonstrated that high levels of job stress are associated with eating and weight gain.

FIRST THINGS FIRST

Before trying to figure out how to break the relationship between job stress and weight gain, the first step is to understand stress itself. In the clearest and most concise terms, it's the emotional and physical reaction that you experience when the demands and requirements of a situation exceed the physical, mental, personal, or other resources that you're able to mobilize. When the demands are high, and your ability to exert control is low, you're going to experience stress. Sources of stress are called "stressors," and the most common place today where you'll find them is on your job.

While stress can wreak havoc on your mind and body, it's important to stress one point first. Namely, when stress levels are moderate or low, they can actually have a positive impact, such as by increasing your strength, energy, focus, attention, alertness, motivation, and overall performance. At the same time, when stress levels are high and continuous, as is typically the case with stressors at work, stress can destroy you.

ORIGINS OF THE STRESS RESPONSE

A brief look at the history of stress, starting with your prehistoric ancestors, will help you deal with today's job stress. They experienced stress, but it was intermittent, such as when a saber-toothed tiger showed up at the cave. When this type of threat appeared on the landscape, your ancestors' brains would instantly kick into high gear. The result would be a series of instant brain-based messages that sailed from the amygdala to the hypothalamus to the rest of the body to prepare for "fight or flight" by instantaneously readying the body to either hit the beast or hit the road. Either way, the adrenal glands would respond with a rush of adrenaline into the bloodstream. This would automatically lead to an accelerated heart rate to push more blood to the body's major muscles and vital organs, increased blood pressure, more sweating to keep the body cool, pupil dilation to take in more of the scene, faster breathing to get more oxygen to the brain, heightened sensitivity to sounds, and the release of glucose to help increase the body's power and energy.

As the threat and resultant stress reaction continued, the hypothalamus would release a hormone that ultimately caused the adrenal glands to send out yet another hormone—cortisol. As you'll soon see, this single process is particularly important when it comes to the issue of weight gain and stress.

For our ancestors, once the threat had passed, the stress reaction would subside and stress levels would remain low until the next teeth-baring or club-bearing visitor showed up on the scene. Importantly, for humans of the prehistoric past, stress was intermittent. But that was then. For employees today, job stress is constant, as today's workplaces abound with managers, coworkers, projects, demands, assignments, conflicts, crises, and working conditions that make a saber-tooth tiger seem like a household pet.

The good news is that our bodies were perfectly designed to handle intermittent stress. The bad news is that our bodies weren't designed for constant stress that employees experience in today's jobs. When the body is in nonstop high-stress mode, the stress response doesn't shut off—and this spells trouble. When held at full-speed, the very mechanism that was essential for human survival can now decrease the likelihood of survival.

STRESS AND YOUR BODY, YOUR THINKING, YOUR EMOTIONS, AND YOUR ACTIONS

Job stress needs to be managed not only because it can easily drive you to comfort foods that drive up your weight, but also because of the vast range of collateral damage that it can wreak on you. There's no way in the world that you'd sit back and knowingly let anyone wreck your body, muddle your thinking, mess with your emotions, or misguide your behavior. But if you don't manage stress, it's going to manage you in several distressing ways.

Physical Damage

Research continues to find a compelling relationship between chronic stress and a shocking array of physical problems, such as heart disease, high blood pressure, spasms of the coronary artery which can lead to chest pain or even a heart attack, stroke, tension headaches and migraines, nervousness, sleep disorders, gastrointestinal and digestive problems, accelerated aging, decreased immunity, backaches, asthmatic episodes, tremors, twitches, increased production of cholesterol, breathing problems, vision problems, vertigo, sweating and chills, nausea, weakness, fainting, and hyperventilation that can induce a panic attack and premature death.

And by the way, when your body directs blood to the major muscles and organs, the lesser functions are set aside. As a result, when people are under stress, it's not uncommon to find that their digestion, salivation, tear production, urinary, and sexual functions don't work well—and that can produce even more stress.

Cognitive Damage

Numerous studies show that when people are under the chronic stress typically associated with their jobs, their thought processes are likely to be markedly muddled. The stress you experience can easily contaminate your cognition with waves of confusion, inattention, distraction, forgetfulness, mental lethargy, diminished intellectual curiosity, thwarted creativity, compromised problem-solving, indecisiveness, rumination, and marginal concentration. The mental acumen and acuity that may have been hallmarks of your intellect easily morph into mental mush as a result of the hit that stress puts on your brainpower. This is illustrated in an experiment conducted at the Ohio State University Medical Center which found that the relatively innocuous act of watching scenes from a visually violent movie can generate sufficient stress to hamper an individual's ability to solve problems. Specifically, participants who viewed twenty minutes of a violent war movie demonstrated less mental flexibility than those who viewed twenty minutes of an animated comedy. If watching twenty minutes of a battle scene in a movie can have a detrimental impact on mental agility, think of what can happen to your problem-solving skills when you're not just watching a battle, but in one—all day long. By the way, there's no question that it's easier to engage in unhealthy eating when job stress makes your common sense uncommon.

Emotional Damage

Not only are your mental faculties compromised by stress that you experience on the job, your emotions can be turned upside-down as well. As the stress of your job winds its way through your brain, a broad assortment of negative emotions can be unleashed such as anxiety, apprehension, worrying, depression, touchiness, agitation, irritability, jumpiness, guilt, grief, uncertainty, self-doubt, helplessness, apathy, mistrust, low self-esteem, pessimism, diminished emotional control, moodiness, feeling overwhelmed, and anger and rage. Any of these emotional reactions can easily lead you to engorge yourself on comfort foods. After all, at least you'll find friendship, comfort, and support with a cupcake or donut. While people at work may let you down, these sweets are always ready to make you feel better, happy, and satisfied—at least in the moment. But if you succumb to the pangs for pleasure foods and savor those sweets and treats, you're ultimately destined to be even more stressed because of the impact that this binge is going to have on your bulge.

Behavioral Damage

In addition to driving you to the sweets table, some of the other proven behavioral outcomes emanating from stress include withdrawal and isolation, temperamental flare-ups and outbursts, suspicion and paranoia, restlessness, accident proneness, shirking of responsibilities, insubordination, substance abuse, nervous affectations and mannerisms, aggressiveness, violence, and anti-social behaviors. In fact, researchers at the University of South Australia found that individuals who experience high levels of stress at work are more likely to unleash anger and aggression while driving. Apparently, the stress that builds up on the job needs a release, and the anonymity and protective shield of an automobile provides the perfect vehicle. With job stress at an all-time high, could this be why road rage is such a common phenomenon today?

WHEN CORTISOL CALLS

One of the most compelling behavioral reactions associated with stress is the tendency to engorge oneself. But technically, at the moment your stress response begins and the adrenaline starts to flow, your appetite will initially decrease. But not for long. In prehistoric times, when whatever was causing the stress had subsided, the stressed-out human would then start to calm down and get back to whatever was normal in those spelunking times. This would include doing some foraging in order to get replenished after an encounter with the Neanderthal next door.

This is the time when cortisol really goes to work. Known as the "stress hormone," it stays in your system longer than adrenaline and signals your body to rebuild its food supply after the fight or flight. The most obvious way that cortisol makes this happen is by increasing your appetite. Back in the day, when that saber-toothed tiger was no longer a threat, cortisol levels would drop after re-nourishment. The problem is that in today's saber-tooth workplaces, when one tiger leaves, another arrives. And some don't leave at all. The result is that your stress levels remain locked in high gear, and so does your cortisol production. And so does your appetite.

When humans were truly in a fight or a flight, they'd use up a great deal of energy, often burning through much of their stored fat and glucose. It's cortisol that sends you a message after prolonged stress that you need to rebuild that storehouse of fat and glucose. Further, your body's preference for brownies over broccoli is due to cortisol's push for the fastest sources of energy, namely foods that are high in fat and sugar. Your body doesn't know that the chronic stress that you experience at work doesn't entail much running, thrashing, or smashing on your part, nor does your body realize that today's stress doesn't burn up much fat or glucose. As a result, your body, with its prehistoric programming, figures that when you've experienced stress, you need some fat and sugar right now. This engorging typically leads to an increase in your weight, along with an increase to your midsection, since this is where such fat tends to be stored.

The reality is that humans are naturally drawn to high-fat and sugary foods as a result of stress. In an experiment at the University of Pennsylvania, laboratory mice were stressed out by being exposed to the odor of a predator, and they were then offered their regular food pellets as well as high-fat food pellets. The result is that the mice greatly preferred the high-fat offerings—which is exactly what those predators at work cause you to do.

When you're encountering stress, it's also natural and normal to seek psychological comfort and relief. Today's humans have been programmed from their earliest years to associate comfort with milk and cookies, cakes, ice cream, and sugary treats, all of which bring back positive memories and imagery from happier days. By savoring those sweets, you're reminded of trips to the donut store after a soccer game, heading to the ice cream shop for getting good grades, or going to the bakery as a special surprise from a grandparent. One of the ways to bring back these feelings—and reward yourself when stress builds up—is to eat something delightful that reminds you of those delightful times. Instead of fight or flight, today's reaction is more likely to be fight or bite.

YOUR STRESS MANAGEMENT PLAN

The process of managing stress starts with the establishment of a goal and a businesslike strategy to meet it. The objective should be to successfully, productively, and measurably manage stress on your job, and you'd support this goal with a three-step action plan. First, identify the key sources of stress on your job. Secondly, establish and implement steps to reduce or eliminate them whenever possible. And finally, establish and implement steps to manage the remaining stress that's irreversibly inherent to your job.

SOURCES OF STRESS ON THE JOB

If you're going to manage job stress effectively and prevent it from flipping you into engorgement mode, you need to flip into management mode. After all, if you don't surrender when you face other problems at work, why would you let a problem such as job stress easily overpower you and hurl you toward the sweets table? When it comes to challenges at work, you dig in and strive to analyze whatever the problem might be, followed by developing and implementing a plan to manage it, lessen it, or prevent it. Since that's your standard businesslike approach to handling job-related problems, why abandon it when you experience job-related stress—especially since stress is one of the most serious and potentially damaging job-related problems of all?

Underlying any plan that you develop in this area is a fundamental workplace reality associated with job stress. Namely, every job is going to generate some stress. In fact, if there were no stress at all, there would be no job at all, as garden varieties of stress can actually have a positive impact. But in today's organizations, work is not a walk in the garden, and stress levels are often pushed permanently into the red zone. While individual stress tolerance can vary from one person to another, research has found that the ongoing stress commonly experienced in today's workplaces takes a toll on virtually everyone.

Stress by Design

One of the primary sources of stress at work is the way your job is designed. If you step back and look at your current responsibilities, you can easily identify any number of possible stressors, such as your absurd workload, excessive hours, lack of control, uneven significance of the tasks, extreme deadlines, overly slow or fast pace, excessive physical and mental demands, lack of challenge, myriad obstacles that prevent you from getting your job done, and minimal opportunities to learn, grow, advance or sense achievement, recognition, personal competence, and effectiveness.

Stress by Others

A separate source of stress on your job can be your fellow employees. Starting first with your manager, there's a huge range of behaviors that she can display that instantly cause your blood to boil. In fact, right at this moment, the mere thought of your manager might be enough to trigger a palpable stress response. Some of her actions might include inconsistent, unclear, or conflicting expectations, excessive demands, micromanagement, condescending treatment, arrogance, insults and degrading comments, lack of communication, unwarranted criticism, unethical behaviors, harassment, non-responsiveness, inattention, public reprimands, lack of support, inequitable practices, arbitrary treatment, disrespect, lack of trust, breach of confidentiality, lying, yelling, and bullying—just to name a few.

Also within the realm of fellow employees who qualify as stressors, it's important to include the rest of your coworkers. Their stress-inducing behaviors know no bounds and can include such antics as arguing, stealing your ideas, nonstop talking, bragging, nagging, complaining, interrupting, pestering, ostracizing, breaching your trust, breaking commitments, failing to listen, nosiness, arrogance, and blaming.

Stress by Yourself

Not only are interpersonal conflicts a significant source of stress, internal conflicts within yourself can be just as stressful. For employees who sense that they're in over their head, in disagreement with the philosophy or actions of the company, or sense that the company is steering their careers in the wrong direction, an internal conflict rages, and this further contributes to raging levels of stress.

Stress by Climate

Another major source of stress on the job emanates from the company's culture, atmosphere, and structure, especially when employees are regarded as replaceable objects that fill slots on the organization chart. Particularly gripping stress inducers are corporate cultures premised on minimal interest in employee ideas and input, one-way communication, inequitable programs and policies, keeping employees in the dark on major changes that impact their jobs and futures, constant change, lack of interest in work/life balance, nonexistent or nonoperational procedures to deal with improper treatment of employees, and a lack of opportunities to learn, grow, achieve, and advance.

Stress by Working Conditions

A further key source of stress for today's workers is the physical workplace. While stressors associated with working conditions are more apparent in inherently risky jobs such as roofers, tree trimmers, and miners, working conditions actually generate significant levels of stress across the full spectrum of occupations. In this regard, some common stressors include loud noise, cramped or crowded work areas, noxious and obnoxious smells, extreme temperatures, uncomfortable or ergonomically dysfunctional furniture, dangerous layouts, and inadequate or inoperable supplies and equipment. While toxic fumes are a clear and obvious danger that has all the earmarks of a stressor, other less devastating nasal assaults can generate equally compelling stress reactions. You can probably remember and even re-experience some of the stress that you sensed when your coworker's perfume overpowered the entire department, or the dank wharf-like odor that wafted through the break room when some of your fellow employees reheated last night's fish, or even the close-talking coworker whose passion for onions brought you to tears.

One of the newest stressors emanating from working conditions today is email. The ongoing barrage of messages can interrupt your work, break your train of thought, and add extra disarray into your already hectic workday. In fact, in a study conducted at the University of California, Irvine, one group of IT employees continued to read their work email, while the second group didn't. Members of the non-email reading group reported that they felt less stress and were better able to stay focused and handle their job responsibilities than members of the email reading group.

RESOURCES FOR DEALING WITH SOURCES

With the sources of stress out in the open, you're in a great position to break the link between job stress and gaining weight. While it's easy to seek comfort foods when you come face-to-face with these stressors, the healthiest and most productive response is to focus your actions on lessening such stressors and even eliminating them. If you say nothing, you're guaranteed to experience more of the same outrageous stressors, followed by more outrageous stress, all leading to outrageous weight gain.

Act Assertively

The key word that lies at the heart of dealing with stressors is assertiveness. This means standing up for yourself in situations in which you have a right to be heard. It doesn't mean acting aggressively or angrily, but rather taking a strong, positive, and affirmative stance on matters of true importance to you. When you encounter stressors on the job, regardless of the source, one of the most productive and effective reactions is assertiveness.

Perhaps you're encountering one of the more common stressors in today's corporate jungle—the manager whose behavior is premised on bullying, harassing, haranguing, insulting, degrading, ignoring, or dominating others. Rather than rolling with his punches, play the assertive card. Meet with him and follow a basic assertive model in which you specify the issues or behaviors that are generating stress, clearly express the way that you feel about these factors, provide suggestions and strategies to deal with them, spell out the possible costs if they continue, as well as the measurable benefits associated with your ideas. This should be a businesslike dialogue—not a complaint fest. If this doesn't lead to some improvements on the stress front, head up the corporate ladder.

Why would anyone in management want to listen to your concerns about job stress and stressors? If your employer is interested in increasing productivity, reducing errors, controlling turnover, reducing absenteeism, harnessing insurance premiums, improving morale, increasing job satisfaction, reducing the number of employees on stress leaves, strengthening employee engagement and commitment, reducing accidents, reducing legal liability, and building employee wellness, you should have no trouble making yourself heard.

Join Forces

If you're concerned about going out on a limb by stepping up and indicating to your supervisor or company management that a certain colleague or job component is generating a high degree of stress, one highly effective way to deal with this matter is to team up with a posse of coworkers. When faced with factual data and suggestions from a credible cadre of employees, employers are more likely to listen. In the case of abusive managers, employers are not only more inclined to take action to deal with them and the stress that they generate, employers don't want to hire them in the first place—a fact evidenced by the growing number of companies specifically stating in their recruitment ads that they don't hire bullies, troublemakers, or jerks.

Management Steps

If you're in management, you can proactively reduce stress levels from every source by keeping an open door and open mind, managing by wandering around, holding formal and informal group discussions, periodically conducting employee surveys, educating employees on stress management and prevention, listening to the employees' concerns, ideas, and suggestions, and implementing a targeted plan of correction. Management often finds that when employees are given an opportunity to express their thoughts about job stressors, they typically deliver an earful. Participating in this type of dialogue often has a cathartic impact for the employees, since the very act of voicing concerns about stressors in hopes of reducing or eliminating them can actually help reduce stress levels.

MANAGE STRESS BEFORE IT MANAGES YOU

At this point, it's time to take action to manage the residual stress that's inherent to your job. Think of stress in the same way that you think of your toughest competitor. That competitor wants to bury you, and so does stress.

This means that you should put yourself at the highest level of personal alertness regarding the stress that you experience. The instant you sense that you're going into stress reaction mode, you need to shift into stress management mode. You're probably familiar with the importance of staying ahead of the curve when it comes to dealing with pain, knowing that failure to act immediately when pain strikes is only going to make it that much more difficult to control with the passage of time. This same concept applies to dealing with stress. If you want to prevent the destructive and debilitating impact of stress, you need to take action immediately, lest you fall behind the stress curve and most likely fall behind in several other ways as well.

People have different reactions to stress, and in order to be a successful stress manager, you'll need to continuously sharpen your sensitivity to all of the early warning signs which indicate that your stress levels are trending upward. As a result, keep an eye out for the first signs of your own adverse emotional or mental reactions, problematic physical reactions, and/or changes in your behavior—any of which can be a tip-off that stress is starting to push you to your tipping point. Be extra vigilant regarding your eating practices—one of the most obvious reactions is that employees who are stressed out tend to pig out.

PROVEN TACTICS TO TACKLE STRESS

For all of the stressors that are irrevocably part of your job or unrelentingly ensconced in your workplace, there are proven stress management methods that'll help you counteract them and the counterproductive impact they can have on you, your work, your job, your food intake, your health, and your life. All you need to do is look over the menu of stress management methods, test out the ones that appear to be right for you, make a final decision as to those that fit best, and then implement them. At the same time, as with any managerial practice, it's important to periodically evaluate the effectiveness of the strategies you've selected and make any necessary tweaks or changes along the way.

Take a Deep Breath

When under stress, one of the normal reactions is shallow breathing, but this is actually the exact opposite of what you should be doing. One of the most powerful ways to bring your stress levels down is through deep breathing. The idea is to slowly take a deep breath through your nose, hold it, and then slowly let the air out through your mouth. This has been proven to lower blood pressure, reduce the heart rate, and decrease many of the problematic mental and physical reactions associated with stress. The American Institute for Stress indicates that this simple and free action is highly effective in reducing anxiety and stress—it helps people relax, calm down, and focus.

In Meditation Mode

Just a few minutes of meditation a day can do wonders when it comes to reducing stress, anxiety, and tension, thereby bringing you to a relaxed, calmer, and more peaceful state of mind. Most forms of meditation involve deep breathing and focused attention on one item, whether it's an object on your desk, an image in your mind, or even your own deep breathing. The overall idea is to sit tall and comfortably, close your eyes, relax each part of your body from head to toe, breathe slowly and deeply, and even repeat the same word or phrase softly to yourself. While there's obviously far more to meditation than these rudimentary steps, even the most basic forms can be powerful stress reducers.

The Exercise Factor

Another highly effective way to reduce your stress is by exercising. Whether it's through frequent visits to the gym or by engaging in regular informal exercises on your own, there's no question about the power of exercising when it comes to stress management. In fact, according to the Mayo Clinic, exercise of virtually all types, including yoga, jogging, aerobics, or any other activities, can play a major role in managing stress. Research continues to find that exercise lessens fatigue, releases mood-enhancing endorphins, improves mental awareness and focus, clears your head, builds your self-esteem and self-confidence, helps you sleep, and even strengthens your problem-solving skills.

Walk It Off

When stress starts to build up and you feel it percolating with each passing minute, get up and walk around. By hitting the bricks, you can take advantage of several stress-reducing techniques at once. This includes extricating yourself from a setting that's generating the stress, clearing your thinking and gaining a new perspective, capitalizing the health benefits associated with walking, and even doing some light meditating along the way. As was found in a study conducted at the University of Georgia, sedentary individuals who expressed frequent concern about their fatigue increased their energy levels by 20 percent and decreased their fatigue by 65 percent as a result of regular low-intensity exercise such as walking.

Write It Out

Another powerful strategy to help subdue job-related stress is to sit down with a sheet of paper and write out exactly how you feel about whatever's getting you so stressed out. Spell out the distressing elements in detail, along with the full range of emotions that you're experiencing. The idea is to release all of your feelings. As reported in *Advances in Psychiatric Treatment*, writing about stressful events can lead to improvements in physical and psychiatric health. One of the key long-term outcomes of this technique was that individuals who engaged in this written catharsis had fewer trips to the doctor for stress-related matters. When stress levels build, it's important to let them out. Going back to the pen and paper may be "just write" for you.

Stress Mitigation by Affirmation

One of the more innovative ways to manage stress effectively is based on studies that deal with positive affirmations, namely strong and empowering messages that you give to yourself—through a personal pep-talk or a silent verbalization and confirmation of some of your deepest values and beliefs. Researchers at Carnegie Mellon University found that one way to counteract the negative impact that stress has on creative thinking is through affirmative statements. The act of frequently giving yourself positive messages such as, "I keep cool under fire," "My resilience is remarkable," or "I thrive when the going gets tough," has the power to reduce the debilitating impact that stress can have on your thinking and problem solving. Rather than letting the stress of the job turn your problem-solving skills into a problem, give yourself regular self-affirming messages throughout the day and even as you're falling asleep at night.

Cut the Clutter

Another way to get a leg up on stress is to remove the clutter from your work area. The vast assemblage of files, documents, trinkets, and chotchkies that you've accumulated over the years are all contributing to the stress that you're experiencing on your job. If you cut down on the clutter, you'll cut down your stress. Clutter generates stress in several ways, such as by making it difficult for you to find what you need when you need it, sending a worrisome message to you that you don't really know how much work awaits you in the piles of documents on your desk, and preventing you from really knowing when your work's done. If you want to avoid being swamped by clutter, start tossing excess papers, files, documents, and uncollectibles overboard. If your desk looks like an archaeological dig, you can easily be perceived as a dinosaur, especially in today's world of electronic documents and reduced reliance on paper. Find a space for everything that you need, and then donate, recycle, or trash the rest. At the end of each day, put the remaining items where they belong—this will help get your stress levels to where they belong.

Perhaps a Nap

Although the traditional work ethic may frown on the notion of naps, often placing them in the terminable category of sleeping on the job, a brief nap is actually another powerful way to reduce your stress. Also called a power nap, it's a brief stint of shut-eye lasting around twenty minutes that you'd grab during the day. Research on power naps has consistently found that they not only reduce stress, but also improve the napper's memory, creativity, productivity, ability to focus, energy, and general state of mind. In addition, sleep researchers at NASA found that a brief nap of twenty-six minutes can increase performance by 34 percent. Add to this the finding of researchers at the Salk Institute for Biological Studies who determined that a brief nap actually helps brain activity stay at a high level all day, and the prospect of some sanctioned shut-eye becomes more appealing.

Progressive Muscle Relaxation

When you're under stress, one common outcome is that your muscles become tense and tight. While this is appropriate if you're in fight-or-flight mode, it can be debilitating and even dangerous for you to remain in this state for prolonged periods. When your muscles are knotted up, your stress levels are likely to be up as well. You can help relieve such stress through what's called progressive muscle relaxation. The idea is to sit in your office or a quiet area of your workplace, and after a few deep breaths, tighten and relax each muscle group—beginning with your feet and working your way up. While the impact of this type of conditioning isn't instantaneous, you're likely to find that your ability to relax and manage your stress will become progressively better as you practice. This technique also helps you gain increased understanding of the way that stress impacts the muscle groups throughout your body. This heightened awareness can serve as an early warning system to let you know when stress is building up, thus enabling you to take prompt action to stay ahead of the stress curve.

Valuing Voluntarism

There are plenty of excellent reasons to engage in volunteer work—satisfaction that comes from helping others, giving back to the community and society at large, supporting a cause that's particularly special to you, meeting new and interesting people, and engaging in an activity that's genuinely significant, appreciated, and meaningful. And further, studies have found that when employees engage in volunteer work, their stress levels decline. In one such study, 78 percent of the participants who engaged in volunteer work responded that it lowered their stress levels. Voluntarism is truly a "win-win-win" situation, as society, employers, and employees all benefit from this single practice. In fact, growing numbers of companies are recognizing and acting on the benefits associated with voluntarism. This support comes in many different forms such as providing employees with paid time off to do volunteer work. If you're looking for a way to do some good for yourself when it comes to managing and reducing your stress, you're likely to find it by doing some good for others.

Picture This

Another highly effective way to manage your stress is through guided imagery. Based on using your imagination, guided imagery is a way for you to take yourself on a mental journey to a real or imaginary favorite spot. Numerous studies have found that guided imagery leads to measurable reductions in stress. With your eyes closed, picture yourself in your happy place and see yourself doing something you enjoy, whether it's reading, playing tennis, body surfing, hiking, or just kicking back. Bring all of your senses into play—focus in detail on the sights, sounds, smells, tastes, and tactile sensations that characterize this special place. Hear the birds chirping. Feel your feet sinking in the billowy sand. Breathe in the pristine air. Stay there until you feel yourself relaxing, and then open your eyes, take another deep breath, and return to whatever you were doing before this odyssey. When you feel that the stressors are getting the best of you, try a mental vacation with guided imagery as your guide.

But Wait—There's More

The menu of stress management techniques is obviously vast, and it's the only menu you should look at when cortisol knocks on your door. While some of following additional techniques may not lend themselves as readily to the workplace and its environs, they certainly can be tried at home. They include spending time with your pet, taking a vacation or staycation, practicing mindfulness, watching a funny TV show or movie, getting a massage, using aromatherapy, taking more time to pursue your hobby, listening to soft and soothing music, getting acupuncture, trying self-hypnosis, and talking out your feelings with a friend, clergyperson, or counselor. While stress can definitely push you to the office trough, you definitely have the power to push back.

Chapter 8

Traveling without Unraveling

Your flight's confirmed. Your carry-on's packed. You even bought the travel-size toothpaste. You've finalized the agenda for the meeting. The materials that you shipped ahead have arrived. It would appear that every aspect of your business trip has been mapped out, and you're good to go. Whether you're a road warrior or an infrequent flyer, you know that when it comes to business travel, the last thing you need is a surprise. Yet, surprisingly, one major component of so many business trips is left unplanned—the food.

Airports and train stations are not only packed with busy travelers, but also packed with a plethora of food options just waiting to completely destroy your weight loss plans and goals. With bushels of burgers, dazzling donuts, tons of tacos, and sinful cinnamon rolls, it almost seems impossible to avoid the tempting treats. It's as though the food calls out to you. And why wouldn't it? You can't bring a platter of steaming hot beef and broccoli, orange chicken, and fried rice into an airport, and food is hardly served on planes anymore, unless you count the tiny bag of half-broken pretzels or the soggy ham and cheese sandwich available for purchase. Airport vendors know that it's much easier for you to just grab something inside the terminal and eat it on the plane. Or if you've arrived early enough to have some downtime before your flight, or if you have some leeway during your layover, you can sit down at one of these eateries and grab a bite—or several—before you depart, and then continue to munch on a takeout morsel during transit. Plus, if you're traveling alone, no one ever has to know the quality or quantity of what you're eating, and you can indulge accordingly. This is what nutritionists refer to as an "opportunity binge." With no accountability, you can stuff yourself until you're blue in the face because there's no chance of being caught red-handed.

FAST FOOD DAMNATION

It's time to take a look at airports and train stations through a different lens—a lens that focuses on what's really being offered to you. That bacon cheeseburger has over 800 calories and around forty grams of fat. A cinnamon roll can easily roll in at nearly 900 calories and over thirty-five grams of fat. A chocolate shake weighs in at around 700 calories and twenty grams of fat. Would you like fries with that? Or high blood pressure? Or heart disease? Or hours of self-loathing? That would give you something to do when you're onboard, right? At the same time, many of today's airlines are encouraging obese passengers to purchase two seats for themselves, and some airlines are even starting to charge passengers by their weight. This doesn't have to be you.

You know this stuff isn't good for you. You're an intelligent businessperson. You handle challenges and make tough decisions at work all the time. But why does common sense go out the window when you see the fast food window? It's time to manage your eating on the road with the same skills that you use in managing your work. After all, when it comes to your projects, you have objectives, priorities, strategies, and specific measures of performance. You've applied your planning skills to every aspect of your forthcoming trip, except to the most important component—your health. To complete the plans for your business travel, you need to put food into the process. In fact, it should be a high-level priority. While you may be flying coach, it's time to start treating yourself like first class. Your diet doesn't have to be out of control just because you're out of the office.

TRAVEL TIPS THAT WON'T TIP THE SCALES

Consider technology your new best travel companion when it comes to eating on a business trip. You rely on your smartphone, tablet, and laptop for your work, and you can utilize these same devices for your health. Before your trip, go online to the different websites for the airports and/or train stations that you'll be using and take a look at the eateries and shops that are located at the terminals. There are even apps that can provide you with this information. From this point, visit the websites of the listed food spots and check out their menus, especially in terms of nutritional information. With this as a guide, use your business mindset to make a food plan for yourself. This isn't a general statement about trying to eat healthier since that's not a plan at all—just as telling yourself that you're going to work harder on your job isn't a plan. Rather, tackle this just as you tackled a recent major project by mapping out exactly where, when, and what you'll be eating, and document this information by writing it down in advance. After all, a real project plan isn't just in your mind. And the best part is that if you'd like to stop for fast food, go right ahead. But this time, you'll have decided ahead that you'll be eating a less caloric and less fattening item off their menu such as a low-fat vanilla frozen yogurt which has around 115 calories and two grams of fat per half-cup serving. You don't have to deprive yourself. You're simply devising an effective strategy that puts you in a position to make smarter decisions on your trip, just as you seek to do in all other aspects of your job.

Bring Your Own

When creating your eating plan, you always have the option to bring your own foods and snacks to the airport or train station, presuming that you stay within TSA guidelines on the items you select. Many fruits and vegetables such as apples, bananas, pears, and packaged carrot and celery sticks travel well in every respect. They're low in calories, high in fiber, and full of vitamins, minerals, and antioxidants. They can easily satisfy your sweet tooth and provide you with a necessary crunch. Plus, you have the added time-saving benefit of eliminating the need to wait in more airport or train station lines when trying to purchase something to eat. When it comes to carry-on items, not only are these items light, they'll help make you light as well.

But be honest with yourself. If you know the fruit slices from home aren't going to cut it on travel days, that's okay. Just plan accordingly. You don't set yourself up to fail in any other aspect of your job, so don't set yourself up to fail by bringing an apple when it's not going to be enough to keep you from buying a serving of apple pie. Use the same types of strategies that make you successful on the job, and this includes taking reasonable proactive steps that have a high probability of success—and in this case, one such step is to bring something from home that you'll actually want to eat. Trail mix, nuts, and low-fat granola bars are airport-friendly and figure-friendly options. Plus, there are many low-calorie versions of popular chips, cookies, and crackers that are prepackaged and perfect for travel. When you arrive with food that's pleasing to your palate, you'll be less tempted to stop at a shop in the terminal to buy an oversized and overpriced box of candy. As a side note, some other steps that play an important role in your pre-travel planning are literally the steps you take at your next visit to the grocery store or supermarket. Walk around, pick up boxes, and read labels. With a little exploring, you're likely to discover healthier and tasty products that you never knew existed. Your new favorite travel snack may be right in front of you, just like your weight loss success.

THE ALCOHOL ABYSS

As business travelers head for their destinations, they frequently stop at a watering hole or two along the way. Airports and train stations are replete with restaurants and bars proffering every variety of booze. But when you decide to drink up, what's really going up are the numbers on your scale. Alcohol is full of extra calories. Is it worth it? A Long Island iced tea for 529 calories? A margarita for 417 calories? A White Russian for 307 calories? The bottom line is that if you want to drink, you need a plan. There are apps and online sites that easily enumerate the calories in the drinks you prefer. With that information in hand, just use the same good judgment that you'd apply to that project that's sitting on your desk right now. Gather the data. Analyze it. Make your decisions. Implement them. Stick to them. A new way of thinking about responsible drinking is to remember that you're responsible for the extra poundage that's likely to accompany your bar tab. If you're waiting around at the airport and decide to have a brew or two, don't let your waiting around turn into weighting around.

If you're traveling by air, the next opportunity for alcohol-induced poundage occurs when the seatbelt light is turned off. Perhaps you're part of the legions of business travelers who enjoy taking the edge off after takeoff by tipping a drink or two in flight. But the calories in your mixed drink aren't the only problem when you mix alcohol with air travel.

While it's said that a bird in the hand is worth two in the bush, researchers have found that a drink in the air is worth two on the ground. One drink at 32,000 feet is very likely to leave you higher than you bargained for. A related outcome is that your judgment isn't likely to be as sharp which can make it much easier for you to purchase another drink or two, along with some candy and chips—all pushing your calories sky high. Plus, the dry air on planes can make you dehydrated, which can lead to exhaustion, headaches, dry skin and eyes, and respiratory problems. And guess what beverage is highly dehydrating? Alcohol. Combine the two, and you're making it even harder for your body to function, let alone perform at a top level during your trip. According to the Mayo Clinic, severe dehydration can cause seizures, kidney failure, and even death. You get the point. If you're going to drink alcohol in flight, your plan should be one and done. What you really should be drinking is a lot of water to keep yourself hydrated. Another healthy alternative to ward off dehydration is to snack on fruit, which is just one more reason why fruit makes a great carry-on companion.

The Booze Snooze

For many business travelers, in-flight alcohol also functions as a sedative, helping them relax, calm down, and maybe even catch a little shut-eye. But if relaxation is your objective, there are many healthier, cheaper, and more effective methods that won't thwart your weight loss plan, dull your thinking, or jeopardize your health. Try breathing exercises. The simple repetition of inhaling through your nose while counting to four and exhaling through your mouth while counting to four can help you find your center. As you slow down your breathing, close your eyes, feel your shoulders dropping down, your neck relaxing, breathe in, count to four, and slowly breathe out. At the other end of the relaxation spectrum, you should get up and walk. Yes, even on a plane, when the seatbelt light is off, you should take a stroll down the aisle. Not only will this help you unwind, you're burning calories at the same time. Getting up and taking a brief walk also reduces the likelihood of developing blood clots that can result from a failure to move around for extended periods of time.

If you still feel the need to consume something to calm you, put down the martini glass and pick up a glass of milk. It's a natural sedative that also stabilizes nerve fibers in the brain to help you relax and drift into sleep mode. Another great drinkable option is decaf green tea which among its many benefits contains theanine, an amino acid that can help you catch some zzzs. Keep in mind that caffeine can dehydrate and keep you up, so it's a better choice to pass it up. There are also foods that can help you relax, including almonds, bananas, cherries, and whole grain low-sugar cereal. It's a good idea to have some of these palatable palliatives in your carry-on so that you can carry out your sleeping activity. Plus, you can always save money on wine by purchasing WiFi. With the entire Internet and world of apps at your fingertips, you can find relaxation videos, read the news, watch a movie, play a game, or listen to music.

HAVE MONEY, WILL TRAVEL

Another common perk associated with business travel is a per diem—per day—allowance to cover meals. The terms typically stipulate expenditures for meals and other foods will be reimbursed up to an established daily maximum. There's no policy indicating that you must spend every dollar allowed, but for some travelers, this policy means "use it or lose it." In their mind, the goal is to spend as much of this money as possible. The problem is that if your objective is to simply use it, you're not going to be able to simply lose it when it comes to extra pounds. Nonetheless, with the per diem in hand, you may find yourself buying extra items you wouldn't normally order, such as appetizers, alcohol, sides, snacks, sodas, desserts, and so on. The reality is that this mindset can get you into trouble. After all, there's no such thing as a free lunch.

Just because you have the means to eat as much as you can doesn't mean that you should. Rather, with a little businesslike planning, predetermine the possible venues where you'll be eating and look up their menu's nutrition facts in advance. Map out what you'll be having for breakfast, lunch, dinner, and possible snacks by selecting options that are aligned with your weight loss goals. You're not a frat boy stuffing his face on spring break in Cancun to win a free shirt. You're in the real world. Use the per diem money as an invitation to make healthier food choices instead of an invitation to gluttony. If you order an omelet, pay extra for more vegetables and healthy ingredients. If you get a salad, add salmon. If you get a sandwich, don't just ask for chicken—make it white meat chicken. Swap your side of fries for a side of fresh fruit. Order bottled water instead of tap. Make special orders for yourself. It's easily within the range of most per diem rates—thus virtually eliminating the likelihood that your company controller is going to bother you about your meal expenses. Use the per diem to your advantage by being painstakingly particular about your food, just as you're painstakingly particular about your work.

Desiring Dessert

Many business travelers find that dessert on the road is one of the hardest items to pass up. But it's time to face the fact that if there's still room on your per diem, and you opt to dive into that cheesecake as a result, there might not be room in your clothes later. The truth is that you have a wide array of choices when it comes to ordering dessert. First, you can always say no. Don't even let the waiter put the menu on the table. It's only going to be harder to resist if you read what they're serving. Why torture yourself? Don't even save room for dessert. Eat enough during the day and at the meal so that you truly don't want it.

But you can still have your cake and eat it, too. Just make sure that you're having dessert because you truly want it, and not because you have unused dollars on your per diem to buy it. A good test is to ask yourself if you'd be ordering dessert if you were paying for it with your own money rather than the company's. If the answer is yes, then use your per diem money to your advantage. Pay the split plate fee, and split the dessert. This can be with a person with whom you're dining, or you can request that half of the dessert stay in the kitchen. You never even have to see it. This way, you aren't tempted to eat more when you have to divvy it up yourself. How many times have you said that you'd just have a taste of pie but then ended up eating the whole slice? You wouldn't set yourself up to fail when sitting in your office, so why do it when sitting in a restaurant? The bottom line is that refraining from spending all of your per diem money should never be too hard to swallow. In fact, it's money well unspent.

CONVENTIONAL WISDOM

A business convention provides employees with a welcome break from the day-to-day routine of office life. Sometimes held at exotic resorts in Maui or at trendy hotspots in Las Vegas, a convention can provide you with a much needed change of scenery as well as an opportunity to learn, share ideas, network, and see the latest and greatest in your field. But regardless of the industry, all of these gatherings have one element in common—the abundance of food for the attendees.

One of the major components of the convention food fest is the continental breakfast, typically consisting of bagels, cream cheese, pastries, cereals, fruits, jellies, juices, milk, coffee, and occasional hot items such as scrambled eggs, breakfast meats, French toast and pancakes with syrup, and oatmeal. All served as a buffet, a hotel generally leaves the food out for a couple of hours in the morning, and convention-goers can stop by and help themselves—using the word "help" very charitably. More often than not, attendees end up hurting themselves by stuffing their faces with stacks of sausages, mountains of muffins, and a bunch of bagels. How can you enjoy a continental breakfast without turning into a continent? First, use the one plate and one plate only approach. You normally don't need ten plates when you eat at home, so why should a buffet be any different? When people take multiple plates, they typically lose track of the items they've shoveled onto them, as well as the quantity of each. As a result, they end up with a vague idea of what they've put in their mouths and how much of whatever it was. The smart strategy is to stick with one plate and be choosy about every item you put on it.

What are the best choices? Oatmeal, fruit, and eggs should be at the top of your list, while pastries, French toast, and syrup should be at the bottom. You know that fresh blueberries are better for you than a blueberry scone. But you don't have to go totally without—just don't go overboard. Divide things in half, thirds, or fourths. Share with someone else. Since one bagel is basically equivalent to eating four pieces of bread, half of a bagel is worth considering. Also, ditch the juice. Nutritionists frequently contend that there's no need to drink your calories. Instead, opt for unsweetened iced tea, a cup of coffee, or water, and get your calories from food. Plus, there are low-calorie powders and zero calorie drops that you can add to your water that won't add to your weight.

Next, hit the buffet line once, and that's all. Period. Don't get up for seconds, thirds, or fourths. The food you select on your first trip is what you'll be eating for breakfast. Done and done. You don't need to overeat just because there's food all over the place. The hotel puts out a lot of food because there are a lot of visitors, not because you're supposed to eat as though you're many visitors. If it's too hard to sit in the dining area when you finish your meal, get up and go back to your room. Or even better, take a walk. You'll probably find other conventioneers who'd like to do some exploring with you, and this type of informal networking is often one of the major benefits associated with attending these conventions. As part of your planning, you should also try to determine in advance who'll be joining you while you eat, and then set a time to eat together. It's too easy to go down to breakfast by yourself, eat your continental breakfast, only to be joined by other coworkers just as you're finishing.

And then what happens? More than likely, you feel compelled to get up and grab more food because they just started eating. With a little planning, you can keep your continental breakfast under control.

WHEN THE CONFERENCE CALLS

Conferences provide another opportunity for attendees to further expand their expertise and their network—and expand their waistlines if they're not careful. Today's gatherings are well planned, and attendees typically receive detailed registration packets that leave no guesswork regarding workshop topics, expert panels, lectures, and seminars, and times and locations for every session. There's also information on presenters' backgrounds and credentials, descriptions of guest speakers at lunches and dinners, and where and when meals will be served. But as thorough as these materials may be, it's ironic that one piece of information that's vital to every attendee is often missing—what foods are being served? There's no question that a menu has been prepared in advance. The problem is that it's generally not communicated, especially in any kind of detail, until you sit down at the table.

While the conference might provide you with an itinerary, you need to create your "eatinerary." Find out in advance what's being served. After all, if you suffered from a food allergy, wouldn't you check ahead and make special arrangements? This is no different. Your health is on the line, so it's time for you to get online or make some phone calls. Talk to someone in management. You should have no reluctance to ask what's being served and even how it's made. The good news is that you're likely to be pleasantly surprised with the friendliness, openness, and support shown by whomever you contact at these hotels and restaurants. You're living in a low-carb, gluten-free, vegan-oriented era, and there's not much you can say to these folks that they haven't heard before. With that in mind, if they're serving fried chicken, ask to have it grilled. Mashed potatoes? Ask for sautéed spinach. Cake for dessert? Ask for the fruit platter. Don't be afraid to make substitutions. There's no substitution for good health.

Perhaps you believe that requesting vegetarian meals for the duration of the conference will keep you in the clear. While this idea has fine intentions, the risk is that you may be served something just as unhealthy, such as a serving of fettuccine alfredo for 415 calories and seventeen grams of fat. The bottom line is that even if you ask for a vegetarian meal, make sure you know exactly what you're getting. A warm vegetable dish with goat cheese and a balsamic reduction? Yes. A chili relleno with refried beans and sour cream? No.

GET BACK WITH YOUR EX . . . ERCISE

Once you've figured out the food situation for your business trip, convention, or conference, it's time to move on to the next component of on-the-road weight control—exercise. For many business travelers, it's hard to find adequate time for a decent workout routine. But when something's hard on the job, does that mean you can't do it? Of course not. If you approach weight loss with the same attitude, you'll find a way to exercise. First, call or check online to see if your hotel has a fitness center or exercise room for guests. Next, look at the conference schedule and map out the times for you to fit in a few trips to the gym—especially if you want to fit into that new business suit. By looking ahead at the conference schedule, you're likely to find some down times such as before the continental breakfast and after the last session of the day prior to dinner—these are ideal slots for workouts. Even if it's only fifteen minutes on the treadmill, a little walk goes a long way. Don't feel that if you can't devote a great deal of time to exercising, then it's not worth doing at all. Newsflash! It's always worth doing. Besides, you're probably not training for a triathlon and in need of an eight-hour workout—you just want to elevate your heart rate and burn some calories.

Hitting the Trail

There are other options besides hitting the gym. Put on your shoes and walk around the hotel. Take a stroll through the grounds. Some hotels even have jogging paths and hiking trails that you can use. To make your walk a little more interesting, ask a coworker or a new friend from the conference to accompany you. It may surprise you to see how many others will want to join in. As part of your walkathon, an additional option is to ask the concierge what's happening near the hotel. Is there a path you can take that'll lead you to an outdoor market? The town square? Some specialty shops and boutiques? If the distance to one of these venues is substantial, you can always walk there and arrange for a car from the hotel to pick you up when you're done—or just hop in a cab or use an app to request a ride.

Pooling Your Assets

Another great exercise option is the swimming pool. Taking a few laps and treading water are terrific low-impact strategies to burn calories, tone your muscles, and fire up your cardiovascular system. It's okay if you're not in training to swim the English

Channel. Simply making the effort is half the battle. Hold your nose and jump in.

Room to Move

If you still don't think you have time to get out and work out, you can always exercise in your hotel room. Do a few sit-ups. Some lunges. Ten push-ups. How about jumping jacks? Switch on the TV and lift two water bottles as weights. If you have access to WiFi, you can find a short yoga or home Pilates video and do some stretching on the floor. Your work calls for some creative thinking, and if you can do it on the job, you can do it off the job. Stop the excuses and start the exercises.

PARTY ON

When the long day of tutorials, discussion groups, and poster sessions has drawn to a close, many conference attendees make their way to an evening event. Drinking. Dancing. Barhopping. Clubbing. No matter which options are selected, when the sun goes down, things inevitably heat up. Consuming alcohol during these hours is often standard operating procedure. But aside from alcohol's added calories, added harm to your body, and added detriment to your weight loss goals, there's a work-related reason why you should predetermine how much alcohol you'll be consuming during these post-conference activities. Without doing so, it's too easy to get caught up in the moment, with one drink leading to another. As your alcoholic consumption and caloric intake increase, your good judgment and common sense decrease. In this world of social media, your updates, photos, videos, tweets, and texts can last forever. The people around you are your colleagues—not your college buddies. Before taking that extra drink and engaging in some goofy or unseemly behavior, ask yourself how you'll feel if your actions have gone viral before you even hit the continental breakfast. Do you really want a video uploaded of you bathing in the hotel fountain? A little planning, forethought, and maturity can help you keep your weight intact—and keep your job intact, too.

Just like on the job, you've got some important decisions to make. As you know from work, the best time to make such decisions is well in advance of the crunch. Decide beforehand what you're going to order and how much you're going to drink. You can't take back what happens if your drinking gets out of hand—there's no app for that. If a few drinks may open your floodgates and release a barrage of insults, gaffes, and love confessions, or put you in a position where you're mindlessly stuffing yourself with mini sliders, chili cheese fries, and onion rings, your plan is clear—it's either no drinks or a one-drink maximum. If your coworkers give you grief about not drinking as much as they do or not drinking at all, you can always order red wine and keep the glass close for as long as you want. You don't even have to drink any of it. As a related option, instead of spending your time agonizing about alcohol, make your way onto the dance floor and have a blast. When you're dancing around, you're burning calories. Instead of getting your drink on, get your sweat on.

WINNER TAKES ALL

Whether you're the top sales representative in your region, part of a sales team that surpassed its goals, a customer service standout, or a collector who's led the way in reducing receivables, some companies reward employees with cruises and resort vacations based on reaching or surpassing specific performance goals. If you're the winner of an all-expenses-paid cruise for your outstanding work, you should be proud of your accomplishment and the recognition from your employer. But there's a caveat—just because you feel like the top dog around the office, don't let your trip bite you in the butt.

Cruise Control

While cruises may take you to far-off places and exciting destinations, they also help passengers cruise their way to obesity. It seems that many of today's cruise liners are nothing more than floating upscale cafeterias. You have complimentary three-course dining and buffets, tapas bars, and pubs all beckoning you to partake, along with specialty restaurants such as steakhouses, sushi bars, and Italian trattorias. As if that's not enough, you have access to different drink packages such as endless soda or endless spirits for the entire cruise. While eating and drinking appear to be at the heart of cruising, you won't be doing your heart, health, or waistline much good if you succumb to the onslaught of seductive food and beverage offerings.

One basic strategy to turn your cruise into a weight loss success instead of a weight gain mess is to continuously remind yourself how you earned this trip in the first place. You won it by setting goals and working extremely hard to reach them. Apply this same level of drive, focus, and commitment to controlling your weight. You'll need to prepare yourself for the edible onslaught that you're about to encounter. When you're cruising, you'll find food at every turn. From the second you wake up all the way to the chocolates on your pillow at night, you'll be looking at food, and it'll be looking at you. Many cruise passengers embark on what's referred to as a "see" food diet. This means that when people see food, this visual cue makes them suddenly want it. It doesn't matter how full they are. Or what time it is. Or what they've already eaten. If it's there, they want it. But this doesn't have to be you. You're not a toddler. You don't suddenly want something just because it's in front of you or someone else is having it. You know your plans and goals, and your job has shown you how important it is to keep them in the forefront of your mind. That type of thinking applies on land and sea.

Cruise and Choose Wisely

When it comes to eating on the cruise, the trick is to not go overboard. Instead, take advantage of the opulent offerings that surround you and make them work for you—not against you. Take full advantage of the omelet bar. Pile your salads high with vegetables plus fresh turkey straight from the carving station. Eat the most perfectly grilled fish prepared to your personal liking. As for alcohol, if you truly can't go without, have an amount that stays on plan. And in the dessert category, cruises have an abundance of unique and exotic fruits you can't find in many other places such as star fruit, persimmons, and quince. These are sweet substitutes if you're looking for something sweet.

Shipshape

Aside from the lavish eateries and decadent dining establishments, cruises also boast equally exquisite fitness centers and spas—and they belong in your plan. You can meet with a trainer and lock in some exercise sessions. With crystal-clear pools, multiple tennis courts, state-of-the-art gymnasiums, and signature saunas, use your well-earned time off to relax, recreate, and rebuild. By doing so, you'll return to your job reenergized, reinvigorated, and ready to work—and ready to win again.

You alone hold the ticket to design and implement the best strategies to manage your weight while simultaneously managing your business travel. When you're on the road and dealing with these weighty matters, you're the captain.

Chapter 9

Conventional Strategies for Unconventional Jobs

As workplaces have changed and evolved throughout the decades, so too have the types, locations, and demands of so many jobs today. They've become as unique as the individuals who do them. Working from home. Working the night shift. Working in food services. And so many more. But as diverse as these jobs are, they all can put you directly in line with a barrage of challenges and consequences that contribute to weight gain.

At first glance, it may be unclear how jobs that don't fit into the typical office mold can mold your body into a bigger size. After all, it seems like many weight gain contributors such as break rooms bursting with baked goods, catered company celebrations, lunch-and-learns, and the peer pressure of pushy coworkers are avoided. But don't be fooled. Time spent in your home office can translate into time spent in your home's kitchen. The night shift can shift into an all-night binge. Just because you're not housed in a traditional corporate environment doesn't mean you're not at risk for committing a corporate sin against your health. Whether you're a freelancer, a neonatal nurse, a café cook, or a person who holds any other relatively unconventional position, you can find yourself eating because you're alone, bored, tired, stressed, depressed, anxious, upset, trying to stay awake, or because tasting food is literally required in your line of work. But what about eating because you're actually hungry? For many working people, that's become the hardest job of all. Fortunately, there are proven strategies to combat the potential poundage that emanates from these types of positions.

WHEN YOU'RE WORKING AT HOME

Working from home has become far more prevalent in recent years. In 2012, approximately 13.4 million Americans worked from home, which is about four million more than in 1999. With advancements in technology, meetings that used to be held in person can now be held via video chat. Face-to-face conversations have been replaced by emails, phone calls, and texts. The need for a centralized office location is becoming more obsolete as companies can easily rely on communication technologies to reach their business associates, customers, and vendors. Technology has also opened the door for many entrepreneurs, freelancers, and independent contractors to run their own businesses and online ventures right from the comfort of their homes.

Another reason for the rise in at-home workers is the economy. Many employers are seizing the opportunity to lower general costs and reduce overhead by having employees work offsite. Even the government has hopped on the work-from-home bandwagon, as the number of employees working at home between 2000 and 2010 increased by 88 percent for federal workers and 133 percent for state workers. According to the Census Bureau, a driving force behind this change was the reduction in costs associated with office space and real estate.

Telecommuting Pros

For many telecommuters, working from home has definite perks. First, the commute is entirely eliminated. That means no more time wasted going to and from work and no more money blown on gas, additional car maintenance, bus passes, train tickets, and the like—the unhealthy aspects of prolonged sitting in transit are left behind as well. Further, it's been shown that telecommuters are less stressed than their commuting colleagues who have to fight the traffic and congestion of daily travel. It's also been found that employees who work from home feel a greater sense of autonomy, control, and satisfaction with their jobs, and telecommuting has also been linked to a better work/life balance. In addition, telecommuters tend to enjoy the freedom and flexibility of working in their own environments. And speaking of environments, working from home also benefits the planet. With less people on the roads, there are fewer emissions of greenhouse gasses.

Telecommuting Cons

But in many cases, the benefits of telecommuting can be full of hot air. Teamwork, solidarity, and creativity can all suffer as a result of business discussions and meetings that lack in-person and hands-on collaboration, feedback, and follow-up. Efficiency can also decrease, as hours and even days can be wasted sending files and documents back and forth, just waiting for responses and approvals from various coworkers that could quickly be obtained face to face. Email itself can lead to a multitude of misunderstandings and misinterpretations, since tone, clarity, urgency, and humor often don't come through when an email pops into your inbox. Further, employees who lack the opportunity to telecommute can feel resentful toward coworkers who are allowed to do so. It's not uncommon for a schism to arise between commuters and telecommuters, and when relationships between employees go south, so can productivity.

Alone at Home

In addition to these work-from-home woes, the most detrimental downside has to do with your health. There are numerous traps and pitfalls that cause working at home to work against your weight loss goals. A major offender in this war with your waistline is loneliness. Many home-based workers have minimal daily human contact. Whether it's an in-person conversation with a colleague or a nod of approval from a supervisor, telecommuters often miss out on common workplace interactions by spending hours of the day by themselves. Without these types of connections and feedback, you may start to feel isolated, alone, and depressed—the perfect recipe for weight gain. After all, humans are biologically social creatures, and instead of being able to reach out to coworkers, you're likely to fill this void by reaching out to candy bars.

Unwanted Ennui

Another component of work-at-home weight gain has to do with boredom. Freelancers and home-based individuals often have unpredictable schedules that vary depending on projects, clientele, and the calendar year. With this type of work structure, you can end up having chunks of time with less to do. And with little on your plate, you may find yourself filling an actual plate in order to pass the time. Plus, when you combine this downtime with the lack of daily interactions and personal contact, you're even more likely to employ yourself with eating. More broadly, even the busiest telecommuters may experience boredom every now and then. In fact, you can get bored whether working at home or in a traditional work environment. That's just the reality. The difference is that when you're working offsite and out-of-sight, you can counter your boredom by occupying yourself with eating—no questions asked.

The Kitchen Beckons

While they say the bathroom is the most dangerous room in a house, when it comes to telecommuting, the kitchen actually takes the cake. Imagine going to work each day with the entire contents of your refrigerator and pantry at your fingertips. How easy it would be to take a few of your daughter's cookies? Or a slice of last night's lasagna? Or a handful of your room-mate's chips? Before you know it, you've eaten the entire bag, and you feel anything but chipper. What's troubling for many telecommuters is that they can't escape the numerous goodies that are only a few steps away. It's just too tempting. And with nobody watching, you can eat whatever you want, as much as you want, for as long as you want, and whenever you want, without any judgment or fear of getting caught. You can stand in front of your freezer eating from the gallon of ice cream, or you can come back to the fridge every hour and graze like a cow. Without the supervision and discipline that one feels in a typical office setting, telecommuters can end up supersizing themselves.

HEALTHY TELECOMMUTING TACTICS

How do you avoid work-at-home weight gain? A fitting tip is to dress the part. A mistake that many telecommuters make is that they don't change out of their pajamas or sweatpants since they're not going into the office. But staying in loose-fitting clothes and stretchy pants will only set you up to stay in lounge mode instead of work mode, and your focus shifts from job stuff to stuffing your face. But by changing into business attire, you're physically and psychologically preparing yourself to act in a professional manner, and you'll be far more motivated to stick to your work and weight goals. Hovering around the fridge and eating uncontrollably will seem far more awkward and unnatural when you're wearing a real suit instead of a sweat suit. Plus, getting dressed will further benefit your mental health by giving you a sense of meaning and purpose, as well as a way to prevent each telecommuting day from turning into Groundhog Day. It's not surprising that a symptom of depression is the lack of motivation to get dressed each morning. Nip this in the bud by making the effort to take on the day like a pro and not a pig—or groundhog.

Marking Your Territory

Another way to prevent telecommuting poundage is to designate a specific work area for yourself. All too often, home-based working individuals end up with files in one room, a computer in the next, and before they know it, everything's disorganized and misplaced, and instead of working like a dog, they're busy trying to figure out if their dog ate their work. While it's not always possible to re-create an office in your home, there are simple steps you can take to make a workspace that's kind to your waistline.

First, don't work in the kitchen. Period. This room contains too many sights, smells, and even sounds that can distract and entice you. The visual cue of a cupcake may be all it takes to lure you away from your laptop. Eliminate this possibility by setting up shop somewhere else. Find a functional, centralized, undisturbed space in your home where you can perform your job effectively— whether this is in a basement or a bedroom. Designate a desk, table, or even a section of a table as your official workstation. By creating as close to a businesslike work environment as possible, you're likely to boost your motivation, outlook, and productivity. It'll also help reduce the daily disruptions and distractions of home life. Further, allocating an office-like space will make it that much easier to stay organized and keep track of the contracts, contacts, receipts, and necessary folders and files that you need for your job. Having a separate work area—even if it's small— will decrease anxiety and the likelihood of a stress-induced binge brought on by the misplacement of important items. It'll also assist with your concentration, efficiency, and weight loss by preventing the need to stop and search for a document, only to end up in the kitchen with a donut.

Staying on Track

An additional telecommuting waist-trimming trick is to create a daily schedule for yourself. Unlike a typical office environment with clearly articulated and interrelated timelines and time-tables, many home-based workers are more able to fly by the seat of their pants in terms of their daily agenda. Unless you want the seat of your pants to keep growing, it's imperative to create a detailed schedule that not only includes timelines and deadlines for your ongoing projects, but more importantly contains the times and contents of your meals and snacks. By predetermining your entire food intake for the day—such as oatmeal for breakfast, an apple for a morning snack, a tuna sandwich on whole grain toast for lunch, a handful of almonds for an afternoon snack, a chicken breast with roasted vegetables and brown rice for dinner, and berries for dessert—you're more likely to stick to this plan instead of foraging around your kitchen throughout the day.

Out and About

Another important aspect of your daily schedule is to set aside a time to go outside. Since it's common for home-based workers to feel isolated, alone, and bored, you can counter these feelings and proven causes of weight gain by planning a time to get fresh air. Not only will leaving your home create an opportunity for much-needed social interactions, studies have shown that the brain produces higher levels of serotonin—a mood-boosting chemical—when you're exposed to sunlight. By going outdoors, soaking up vitamin D, and engaging with others, you'll be improving your state of mind as well as giving yourself deserved time away from your home base. In many cases, taking this time will provide you with a heightened sense of clarity and focus regarding your work and weight loss goals. Schedule a visit to the park. Set up a time to meet with a friend. Bring your laptop to a library. Mix it up and change the scenery so you're not turning to food to spice up your day.

Working-at-Home Workouts

Exercise is also a key step in fighting telecommuting poundage. A great way to approach your scheduled time outside is to go for a walk. Pick a destination for yourself—even if it's to the end of the block—and take a stroll. Exercise releases mood-enhancing chemicals that help fight off depression, which in turn can help you fight off the urge to binge. There are also several home exercise options for you to try, and you don't need fancy equipment or an expensive trainer—many cable providers, websites, and apps have free fitness programs that are great for telecommuters. Plus, there's a huge array of exercise programs that you can use on your video game console. Or you can always turn on your favorite music and dance around your house. That's usually frowned upon in a typical office setting, so use it to your advantage. Taking the time for a workout at home is what makes working at home work out.

SHIFT HAPPENS

Another set of unconventional jobs are those that come alive when most people are sleeping. Welcome to the night shift. While the actual positions that require night shift work are as different as night and day—nurses, air traffic controllers, security personnel, and warehouse pickers and packers—the challenges of working from night until day are all too similar. When your workday is turned upside down, it's difficult to not let that happen to your diet. The good news is that just because you work at night, you don't have to put your weight loss goals to bed.

Night Shift Pluses

Despite the unconventional hours, there are various advantages associated with working the night shift. There are night shift pay differentials, and some jobs require fewer hours for full-time pay. And in some businesses, working at night can put you in a pool with fewer coworkers, and this can ultimately result in less competition when seeking a promotion. Another perk is that working nights can lessen the commute time to and from your job as well as enable you to run errands and attend to personal matters with less people out and about. Depending upon your personality, the night shift can be a great opportunity for those who consider themselves night owls instead of early birds. And that might make you happy as a lark.

Night Shift Minuses

Working the night shift isn't all blue skies. It can take a major toll on your well-being and waistline. Not only is a night shift worker more likely to suffer from sleep deprivation, the disruption to his body's natural circadian rhythm can be particularly harmful. Humans have a built-in internal clock that governs processes such as eating, sleeping, body temperature, and other important physiological functions that can get out of whack when your body wants you to be doing one thing, but you're doing another. Not surprisingly, shift work has been linked to numerous health problems, including gastrointestinal issues, cancer, heart disease, type 2 diabetes, depression, and obesity. Studies have even shown that those who work the same job but merely switch from the day shift to the night shift tend to gain weight. Studies have also proven that food is metabolized differently when one's eating is not in sync with his body's natural clock. Even more clearly, researchers at Northwestern University found that mice that ate during their usual sleep hours gained more weight than mice that ate during their normal waking hours, even though the mice all consumed the same average number of calories. When it comes to the night shift and weight gain, do you smell a rat?

Drowsy Dining

For many night shift workers, eating takes on an entirely new function. Aside from the desire to consume because they're hungry, many of these employees consume in order to stay awake. Eating throughout the shift is a common strategy to ward off snoozing—if you're chewing, you're not sleeping. And you're also hoping that the constant ingestion of food will give you the energy you need to make it through your shift. But this tactic often causes night shift workers to eat a greater quantity of food and take in more calories than would be the case if they were working the day shift. Plus, these late-night eating sessions are compounded by the type of food that's usually available to night-shifters. Unlike their day shift counterparts, night shift workers don't have the luxury of ordering in from the local organic bistro, running down to the cafeteria to grab a salad, or picking up a sandwich at the supermarket during a break. Those places are usually closed. And as every college student knows, what's left are the types of eateries open 24/7, which typically means fast food and pizza. Another popular food dispensary frequented by night-shifters is the vending machine. It's convenient, chock-full of chips, cookies, and candy, and accessible at all hours. Unfortunately, the change spent on these midnight munchies can change the shape of your body faster than you can punch in your selection.

Questionable Quenching

It's not just the less-than-desirable food choices that are a growing concern for night shift workers, but the drink choices as well. Employees are constantly ingesting coffee, tea, sodas, and energy drinks throughout the course of an evening in order to stay awake. And these beverages usually have one thing in common—caffeine. It's common knowledge that caffeine can keep you up, make you more alert, and has long been considered the night shift worker's best friend. But is it? The problem is that too much caffeine can be dangerous. It's a stimulant that affects the central nervous system and can elevate your heart rate, raise your blood pressure, and cause irregular heartbeat, headaches, dizziness, and dehydration. Too much caffeine has also been linked to weight gain and an increased risk of type 2 diabetes. Not such a great pick-me-up after all. When you're chugging down these types of drinks all shift long and night after night, there's really something that needs to be fixed when it comes to your caffeine fix.

Let's Get Personal

An additional cause of night shift worker weight gain is the very nature of the shift itself. These employees often find themselves under a great deal of stress, not only from the demands of the job, but also because their night schedule can disrupt many aspects of their lives. You may be unable to spend quality time with your spouse, go out and celebrate with friends, or pick up your child from school because of your work schedule. This can cause disappointment, frustration, and tension for you and those close to you. To this end, there's a higher rate of divorce among night shift couples, and studies have found that children of night shift employees are more likely to experience symptoms of depression. As a result, it's not uncommon for night shift workers to turn to food in order to help them deal with the stress and strain put on their personal lives by their evening routine. Night shift workers often look to sugarcoat their feelings with actual sugar. Unfortunately, this coping mechanism will only lead to more heartache. When you feel the weight of the world on your shoulders, that weight can soon manifest itself around your midsection.

RIGHTING THE NIGHT SHIFT

How can you prevent the night shift from turning into a big fat nightmare? The first strategy is to make sleep a priority. Sleep deprivation is a very real concern with very real consequences for your welfare and waistline. It's time to apply your business mindset and skill set to create a realistic weekly sleep schedule for yourself, "a bed sched," and stick to it, just as you would any other work-related schedule. All too often, the amount of sleep that night-shifters need and the amount of sleep they actually get are two different things. Due to the necessity to sleep during the day, their much-needed sack-time can be short-lived, interrupted, and take a backseat to other people, priorities, and activities. Designating times, durations, and locations to sleep, as well as setting boundaries which prevent others from disturbing you should be part of your plan. Earplugs, blackout curtains, eye masks, white noise machines, and do-not-disturb signs are small investments that go a long way, and shutting down your phone, computer, and other devices will also help you get shut-eye. The fact is that to prevent putting on the pounds, you need to nourish your body with what it really needs—sleep—instead of fighting off exhaustion with chips, candy, and caffeine. And while weekly bed scheds will be unique to you and your work responsibilities, needs, and commitments, aiming for eight hours of sleep per day is an optimal goal to set. Researchers in the Harvard Division of Sleep Medicine recommended that firefighters nap in the late afternoon before a night shift. Is this always possible? Of course not. But the good news is that you have the power to take charge of your sleep cycle so you won't be desperately turning to food to charge up.

Give It a Rest

Placing sleep at the top of your priority list will also benefit your on-the-job performance. People are far more likely to have accidents and make mistakes at work when they're tired. Research has found that sleeping only five hours per night during a week is the same as going to work with a blood alcohol level of .1 percent. That's equivalent to the blood alcohol level of a 180-pound person chugging five beers! And much like being drunk, a lack of sleep significantly impairs your motor and cognitive abilities. Not only are night-shifters desperately relying on food to combat the sleepiness that may cause errors, the added stress associated with the possibility of having a slipup is another cause of weight gain. But by getting more sleep, you'll be less likely to make a miscalculation or blunder because you'll be more alert, awake, and focused instead of sleepwalking through your shift. Not only will your overall outlook improve, but a clear and attentive mind will also help you make better food decisions. Further, being well-rested will decrease your likelihood of becoming sick. Sleep, wellness, and weight loss are all intrinsically linked. Get the memo.

Night Walking

When it comes to eating on the night shift, if you're ingesting crap all shift long in order to stay awake, the first action is to put down the candy and get up and move around. Walking increases the oxygen in your body, which in turn increases your energy, attentiveness, and concentration. Research has even proven that walking is more effective for long-lasting energy than sugar. Plus, walking gives you the added benefit of burning calories, which is especially crucial for preventing night shift weight gain. By taking the time to walk around each night on the job, you're elevating your heart rate while simultaneously elevating your focus and alertness. If you want to go the extra mile, invite a coworker or two to join you on your stroll. Chatting and engaging with others can help you stay awake. Additionally, the change of scenery can reenergize you and stimulate your brain, and walking in well-lit areas can further give you the boost to conquer weariness.

Night Napping

Another trick of the night shift trade is to find times to nap. Even if it's merely shutting your eyes and resting your head for ten minutes in the break room, this can be just what you need to give yourself a boost of energy. A New Zealand study revealed that air traffic controllers on the night shift performed better on alertness tests after a forty-minute scheduled nap period. Napping has also been linked to higher levels of productivity and employee satisfaction, which is why some businesses now have designated "nap rooms" filled with recliners. Plus, various companies have taken workplace napping to a new level with state-of-the-art ergonomically-designed nap pods that can play calming rhythms to lull you to sleep. Of course, depending upon the progressiveness of your company and their likelihood of purchasing pricey pods, there are other smaller changes such as comfier chairs and quiet zones that can be good options for nap-seekers.

Researchers have also determined that napping can make people more effective problem solvers. And further, napping can help solve the problem of on-the-job lethargy.

Fighting Fogginess

Another food-free strategy to beat night shift fatigue is to put on headphones and listen to pump-up music. Just like a football player before a big game, listening to songs with fast and upbeat tempos can energize you and put more pep in your step. You can also go into the bathroom and splash cold water on your face. And speaking of water, make sure you're frequently drinking it during the course of the night. Being dehydrated can leave you feeling weary and drained, and having a water bottle by your side can quench the desire to down other sugary drinks.

Talk It Out

When it comes to warding off night shift weight gain, it's imperative to communicate with those around you, both at work and at home. If you're in an occupation that requires variable shifts, be vocal about requesting a schedule that has some sort of pattern that facilitates your body's adjustment. Working a haphazard schedule with day shifts and night shifts all scrambled together can end up scrambling your brain. If possible, try to obtain a schedule that aligns with your body's needs and rhythms, such as a week of nights followed by three weeks of days or even permanent night shift work. The more the schedule fits you, and you fit the schedule, the easier it will be for your body to adjust to the changes in your normal sleeping and eating patterns. Plus, you won't have to desperately cling to caffeine, cookies, and crap as a way to get your body into workmode.

Amending the Vending

Communication in your organization also comes into play when looking at your work environment in general. Since a night shift hot spot is usually the vending machine, recommend that the vending machines include some better options—low-fat granola bars, bags of trail mix, and sugar-free candies. You can even suggest supplementing or replacing your company's vending machines with others that offer low-sugar, organic, and gluten-free choices. Stocked with fresh apples, pita chips, banana crisps, and soy milk, these handy and healthier snacks can supplement you instead of sabotage you. Isn't it about time that the food options in your workplace start working for you and not against you?

The Home Front

Be open with your partner, your children, and your friends about your needs. Take the necessary steps to create a home environment that respects your goals, both in terms of your work as well as your weight. If you'd like the house quiet at a certain hour or if you'd like to leave an event early in order to get to sleep at a specific time, be candid and assertive about your needs. You're proactive on the job, so why not here? Honest communication in your home life can help lower your stress level and in turn help lower your weight. The more you bottle it up inside, the more you're going to weigh.

Feeding Time

The next tactic for tackling night shift weight gain is to eat according to the time of day and not according to your shift. A mistake that many night-shifters make is that they eat their larger meals during the late-night and very early morning hours. That kind of planning is only going to pack on the pounds. If it's 6:00 p.m., it's dinner. If it's 3:00 a.m., it's not. It's that simple. Your body will thank you. Plus, by including certain kinds of foods during conventional mealtimes throughout the day as well as having the right kinds of snacks available throughout your shift, you can satisfy your hunger while simultaneously getting the energy and nutrition you need for top-level performance. Night shift employees' main meals should incorporate protein-rich choices such as fish, white meat chicken, white meat turkey, tofu, and eggs—they're powerhouse options to fuel your body and brain. Scientists have proven that protein helps you feel fuller longer, and it can also help keep you focused and alert without weighing you down. Incorporating fruits and vegetables into these meals will also help with successful weight management, as they're packed with fiber that can keep you fuller longer—along with their many other health benefits. In terms of carbohydrate-rich foods such as cereal, rice, and pasta, it's recommended that you avoid overloading on them in order to avoid the drowsiness that carbs can bring later on. Additionally, try to avoid eating a giant meal immediately before the start of your shift. Stuffing yourself with food is only going to make you feel more lethargic shortly after.

Bring the Best

Bringing your dinner with you each night is a time-friendly, figure-friendly, and wallet-friendly meal tip for busy night-shifters. Stop relying on 24-hour eateries and vending machines to make decisions regarding your meals and caloric intake. Do some planning and designate a time to visit your local super-market to stock up on healthy meals and snacks for the coming week that'll nourish and sustain you throughout your shifts. A great choice is to visit the bar—the salad bar, that is. Not only will this minimize the amount of time you need to spend preparing a meal to bring with you, but today's salad bars have become far more upscale and contain far more food options than in years past. In addition to your basic assortment of vegetables such as mushrooms, cauliflower, and broccoli, as well as cooked meats like tuna and chicken, many salad bars contain more exotic ingredients such as kale, seasoned tofu, artichoke hearts, and a wide variety of nuts and seeds. Plus, since you're paying by the pound, you can make the salad bar cost-effective as well as health-effective since many of the items are far more expensive per pound in other sections of the store. Further, by holding off on the dressing, this will lower the weight and cost of the salad and prevent it from getting soggy, while enabling you to choose your own dressing and perfectly control the amount. When selecting a salad dressing, look for the ones which are oil based—such as a vinaigrette—since oils such as olive oil and soybean oil can help your body absorb key vitamins and nutrients from the salad itself.

If you're really in a time crunch and searching for something yummy to crunch, there are also frozen meals that won't put a freeze on your weight loss goals. Look away from the lasagnas, taquitos, and chicken pot pies whose high-fat, salt, and carbo-hydrate content will cause your jaw to drop and your weight to soar. You know that crap is bad for you! Instead, nutritionists recommend frozen meals that contain less than 550 mg of sodium and plenty of fiber. By keeping your choices within these parameters, microwaving can be a hot new way to zap calories.

Once your night shift main meals are established, the next step is to determine beforehand what you'll be snacking on before the candy bar is in your hand. Fruits and vegetables are ideal choices, plus you can enhance them with prepackaged servings of nuts and low-fat cheeses. Yogurt is also a standout snack star, especially with the variety of flavor options, types, and textures of yogurt on the market today. Nutritionists agree that yogurt has numerous health benefits—it's a good source of protein, calcium, and vitamin D, and contains helpful bacteria that are good for your digestive system. Research has also shown that yogurt may even lower your risk of high blood pressure. Plus, yogurt is easy to transport with its built-in serving size in each container.

Caffeine Fiend

Then there's the inevitable coffee conundrum. To drink or not to drink, that is the question. Since too much caffeine can be harmful, the maximum recommended amount is in the range of 400 mg per day, which is roughly equivalent to four cups of brewed coffee. This means real, measurable cups and not that monstrosity from your favorite coffeehouse. Wake up and smell the coffee. And as for chugging any caffeinated beverages, including soda, tea, and energy drinks night after night, just remember that caffeine's a drug. Wouldn't it be nice to not be dependent on it? Your waistline as well as your wallet will thank you. Looking specifically at energy drinks, many brands have been linked to health issues, including chest pain, irregular heartbeat, and even death. Now's the time to start replacing your endless stream of caffeinated drinks with water or decaf low-cal options. At the very least, if you simply must ingest any caffeinated drink, do so at the beginning of your shift—drinking caffeine later in the evening or early morning is only going to make it harder for you to fall asleep when you should.

FOOD, NOTORIOUS FOOD

You can't turn on the television today without stumbling upon reality shows and competitions dedicated to cooking, baking, and/or striving to create the perfect meal, dish, bite, and restaurant. Celebrity chefs all abound with their signature cuisines, styles, brands, and products, whether they're endorsing food companies, cooking utensils, hair products, or even starring as daytime talk show hosts. But behind the closed doors of the kitchen, most food industry employees have bigger fish to fry. How do you avoid putting on the pounds when working with food is your meal ticket?

In the Food Biz

From cupcake bakers to fast food servers to event caterers, there are nearly 13.5 million restaurant industry workers in the United States, and enrollment in culinary school is on the rise. Unlike working in a typical corporate environment, food industry employees encounter a unique on-the-job challenge—they spend day-in and day-out surrounded by food. This means that for many of these individuals, each day at work is a constant weight gain war. The seemingly endless supply of deliciously appetizing sights, smells, and sounds can be an all-consuming struggle when it comes to what to consume. Studies have proven that the mere photo of an enticing delicacy can stimulate hunger. What do food industry workers do when faced with seeing, smelling, hearing, and making the actual delicacies over and over each workday? The display case of donuts. The sizzle of steaks. The scent of snickerdoodles. The kneading of pizza dough. This can be all too overwhelming and ultimately lead to overeating. Food industry workers are in a real pickle.

Additionally, for some members of the food industry such as chefs and culinary school instructors, the necessity to taste particular foods and dishes is part of the profession. How can you judge, alter, improve, approve, disapprove, enhance, or serve something if you don't try it for yourself? That leaves many employees taking bite after bite after bite without realizing how much it's taking a bite out of their weight loss goals. Further, food industry workers are often encouraged to consume the food that's being made in their particular workplace. Many companies provide free and discounted drinks, meals, coupons, and other dining perks and privileges to employees. Aside from the convenience and monetary incentive to indulge, these workers may face the added pressure from supervisors and peers to partake in the food fest. After all, what kind of employee are you if you don't want the food that's being made at your company?

RECIPE FOR SUCCESS

Fortunately, there are several ways to avoid turning into a pig when working with food is how you bring home the bacon. When you're constantly bombarded with the sensory cues brought on by spending your working hours around food, instead of grabbing something to eat, you should first reach for something to drink. What's the best option? It's water, hands down. In fact, you may find that your feelings of hunger brought on by the bombardment of foodstuffs around you just might be feelings of thirst. It can be challenging to distinguish which is which, especially in such an enticing environment. Your first line of defense to put out the hunger fire should be water. If you're not a water worshipper, you can spruce up your cup by adding a squeeze of lemon, lime, or other fruit garnish which can be plentiful in many food industry settings. After downing your drink, do yourself a favor and wait for fifteen minutes. It'll give you time to recognize if you're truly hungry. If you continue to have hunger pangs, these fifteen minutes will also give you the time to refocus on your weight goals and find the appropriate item to eat. Chefs say to let meat rest before you eat it, so give yourself a moment to rest and regroup before you eat. And to top it off, studies have proven that having water before meals can help you lose weight.

Just Bring It

The next weight loss weapon in your arsenal is to turn your food workplace into a BYO. That means bringing your own food with you to work to starve off temptation. Make sure you have go-to low-cal snacks available for yourself, including vegetables and fruits—especially those with high water content such as cucumbers, celery, baby carrots, watermelon, and strawberries. They can help keep you hydrated, fuller, and can satiate feelings of hunger that may be brought on by your workplace's flood of French toast, fried chicken, or fudge bars.

A Matter of Taste

If your job includes tasting food, there are ways to prevent your intake from overtaking your weight loss efforts. First, determine how much you actually need to eat in order to properly judge a given item. You may find that a smaller spoonful, sliver, or sample works just fine. Plus, utilizing a littler utensil to taste the food or dish in question can help reduce calories. Also, trust your coworkers, colleagues, and sous-chefs for honest feedback on the foodstuffs so that all of the tasting doesn't fall on you and weigh you down. Speaking of honesty, it's time to be honest with yourself and recognize how much food you're taking in while working. Those bites can add up, even equaling an entire meal or more. If that's the case, use the BYO strategy to supplement this intake with healthier snacks instead of another giant meal.

Prime Choice Exercises

Exercise is also an essential step in weight management for food industry workers. You can keep making up excuses to avoid it, but do excuses cut the mustard while on the job? Could you ever tell a catering client that you "didn't have time" to bake the quiche appetizers for her wedding or that you were "too tired" to make the chocolate soufflés for his dinner party? Would you say to your manager that you "didn't feel like" folding up the napkins or weren't "in the mood" to wipe down tables? As soon as you think about your exercise excuses in the context of your work, you realize how ridiculous they are. When faced with unpredictable hours and heavy time commitments, get creative with your exercise plan—even if it means running up and down the stairs of the restaurant or lifting bags of potatoes as weights. Every effort you put in counts, and it'll get easier with time.

Perks That Work

Another tip for food industry workers is to use the various dining privileges offered by your employer as weight loss perks instead of weight loss punishments. If you're entitled to free or discounted food items, use a businesslike proactive strategy and channel your initiative, insight, and inventiveness into finding the foods, items, and dishes that align with your weight goals. Ask the kitchen staff at your venue how something is made. Check your company's nutrition information, whether online or in-store, and decide what you want to eat—and not eat—before arriving at work so that the calling of calzones, cobblers, and Canadian bacon doesn't take over. Don't be fooled into downing something unhealthy just because it's free or discounted. You're not stupid. Besides, you know you'll pay for it later in so many ways, so what's the point? Instead of giving in and giving up, you can employ the BYO technique and bring your own food with you. Then you can use the free and discounted items as you see fit so that you can stay fit. If your company offers a grilled chicken but it's on a greasy bun slathered in a fattening sauce, wipe down the chicken and bring your own salad ingredients, such as lettuce, vegetable toppings, and an oil-based dressing of your choosing. Can't stay away from your bakery's sweets? Bring your own yogurt and add the inside fruit layer of a fruit tart or a spoonful of chocolate sprinkles in order to create your own lower-calorie concoction. Use the discounted freebies as a way to enhance your meal and truly get your money's worth. That way, you can partake with your peers without taking apart your weight loss goals.

Wrapping It Up

Another possible weight gain pitfall emanates from the extra items that are sometimes given to food industry employees as gifts at the end of a shift. It's a common scenario—since the food wasn't eaten and can't be served the next day, it falls upon you to take home the extra scones, muffins, and coffee cakes so that they don't end up in the garbage. On the one hand, you don't want to sabotage your weight loss efforts, especially if you foresee yourself giving in to temptation and eating a dozen donut holes on the commute home. On the other hand, wasting copious amounts of food doesn't sit well with you either. The good news is that there's a clear answer to this free food face-off—stop deliberating and start donating. There are plenty of worthy organizations that work with food companies of all sizes to get perishable items into the hands of people who need them. Take action right now to implement this kind of partnership in your workplace so that there's no question regarding what to do with the extra food. Plus, knowing that you're helping others is a kind of satisfaction that no amount of pastries could ever provide.

ATTENTION UNCONVENTIONAL JOBHOLDERS!

To all telecommuters, night shift employees, food service workers, truckers, warehouse staffers, dispatchers, air traffic controllers, security personnel, casino workers, and anyone else who has an unconventional job—it's time to stop using the circumstances of your job as a way to justify weight gain. Guess what? They don't. In the end, it's up to you to commit yourself fully to what you want to accomplish, just as it's up to you to commit yourself fully to what you want to accomplish in your career. Take responsibility. Take control. Take action. And take off the weight. There's nothing unconventional about it.

Chapter 10

Let's Do Dinner

As the hours on the clock pass by, your workday turns into night. But your job continues to put you at high risk for weight gain even after the sun goes down. Whether you're heading home, heading out, or heading into additional hours of work at the office or elsewhere, the evening can present pound-popping challenges at every turn. Many people are so exhausted after work that the mere thought of having to work a healthy meal into their nightly routine is exhausting in and of itself. When you're feeling burned out from a day on the job, the quick and easy food choices are the ones whose calorie counts are anything but quick and easy to burn off. There are also many individuals who need to keep working long into the night, whether they're putting in overtime, staying late to wrap up a project, or continuing to carry out job-related tasks and assignments offsite. It seems there isn't enough time to occupy yourself with eating foods that benefit your weight when you're preoccupied with a deadline that just can't wait. So senseless snacking, disastrous dining, and deferred bedtimes ensue, all resulting in work-induced weight gain.

While a 2013 Consumption Gallup Poll revealed that eight in ten Americans eat fast food monthly with over half who eat it weekly, it may surprise you that more than seven out of ten weekly consumers—or those who eat it more frequently—believe the food isn't good for them. So what's going on? Would you ever consistently do something job-related that was harming you, your coworkers, or your department? Why is there such a divide between your work-life and your weight-life? And in terms of your social life, there are also many working individuals who leave work and head off to happy hours and restaurants, but the food and drinks typically ordered at these venues should give you some serious reservations. Taco Tuesday can turn into Weight-Gain Wednesday if you're not careful. Stop letting that screwdriver screw you. On the bright side, even with all of the potential food pitfalls that may befall you come nightfall, you can prevent this from becoming your weight downfall.

THE DINNER DILEMMA

Dinner has taken a hit, and you can thank your job. One of the central causes behind dinner's demise is that working people today are spending more and more time on and at work. In 2014, the average full-time United States employee reported working nearly forty-seven hours per week, with approximately 40 percent indicating that they worked at least fifty hours per week. So much for the forty-hour work week! And when you throw an unstable economy and job insecurity into the mix, it's clear why your day job has taken precedence over your nightly meal. Since work has become a main focus, your evening main course is just not a main course of concern. To that end, family dinners have also suffered work wounds, as the prevalence of these dinners over the past twenty years has decreased by 33 percent, and the length of family dinners has declined substantially as well.

Besides, who has the time, energy, patience, or even the desire to focus on dinner after a long and hard day at work? With constant pressure, demanding bosses, stressful meetings, long commutes, assignments to complete at home, and more, the list of dinner destroyers goes on and on as your weight goes up and up.

Technologically Speaking

Technology also plays a part in today's dinner downslide since employees are constantly connected to their work assignment, projects, and tasks during their downtime and dinnertime. Your phone, tablet, and laptop keep you on-call and online virtually nonstop. In fact, it's been reported that 80 percent of Americans continue to work outside the office, so much so that employees rack up an average additional hour of work per day—this equals an additional workday each week! That's a lot of extra time on work, and many individuals feel it's simply not possible to allot some of their extra-extra time on dinner. Their schedules are just too tight, which in turn is what's happening to their pants. Distracted eating, engorging on fatty foods, and downing detrimental dinners have become the nightly rituals for numerous workers worldwide. Instead of consuming beneficial foodstuffs, your evening's consumed with completing work stuff for your stuffy boss while you completely stuff your face.

In the Zone-Out

Another dinner deflator and weight escalator is the post-work "zone out." After a hard day at the office, an appealing and popular activity for employees is to mentally check out. You've been on point all day, so what's the point of having to appoint any more mental potency to dinner when you're at the point of exhaustion? A common practice by countless working people is plop themselves on the couch in front of the TV and dig into food. In fact, a CBS News poll revealed that 33 percent of American families always have the television on while eating dinner. But zoning out while you put foodstuffs in can lead to mindless munching. This foul food play can drive your weight straight into the red zone and should be considered an illegal procedure. More often than not, you'll end up finishing that bag of chips, package of popcorn, and pint of ice cream in a comatose-like state without even realizing it. Along those lines, the post-work zone out is also contributing to portion size neglect, as even the most meticulous, diligent, and detail-oriented individuals suddenly seem to cast compulsiveness aside when tracking the quantity of their evening meal.

DINNER WINNERS

The good news is that there are simple switches you can make to put dinner back in the spotlight and keep yourself light in return. The first tip is to refrain from giving any electronic devices a seat at the dinner table, especially since 38 percent of Americans admit to checking their work email during dinner. It's too difficult to keep track of portion sizes and too easy to overeat when your attention is somewhere else. You shouldn't drive distracted, and you shouldn't dine distracted. Put down your phone and pick up your fork. Be present while you eat and give yourself the time to taste and enjoy your meal. Even if you have work to do, emails to send, calls to return, orders to place, reports to review, and projects to finalize, it's time to slow down and sit down so you can down your meal in peace. This type of conscious eating will not only help you be more in tune with your hunger signals and prevent overfeeding, it'll also give you the mental breather you need before approaching any of your evening's job-related tasks. This time away to refuel and replenish can actually recharge your thinking, focus, and creativity.

TV-Free Dining

It's also important to end the post-work zone out once and for all. The bottom line is to get your bottom off the couch and turn off the TV during dinner. Taste your food instead of shoveling it down your throat. Engage with those around you instead of acting like an android. Bring family meals back in vogue, especially since eating as a familial unit has numerous psychological, social, and weight management benefits for your family members. You can watch your zombie shows after dinner—don't let your job turn you into one. While it's clearly important to relax, kick back, and take a load off after work, this shouldn't take place while loading food into your mouth. Stop watching TV and start watching your weight instead.

Downsizing

Additionally, it's key to keep in mind that getting off work doesn't mean you're off the hook when it comes to proper portion size, especially in light of—or in heavy of—today's supersized society. Portion sizes have been wildly increasing throughout the years, and research has shown that today's average adult consumes 300 more calories per day than in 1985. When it comes to eating dinner, it's time to stop becoming portly because of your portions. The first tip is to prevent your plate size from messing up your waist size. As found in a Cornell University study, not only did people eat more when they consumed off larger plates, they ended up underestimating the amount of food they ate and believed they ate less. Talk about getting "manipu-plated." Not only is it better to eat off smaller plates, it's also useful to have a handy portion guide to help eliminate the risk of a plate fake out. Fruits and veggies? The size of your fist. Protein? Your palm. Snacks? Your hands cupped together. Starches? A cupped hand. Cheese? Your thumb length. Giving the middle finger to portion sizes will only get you forked.

Be sure to employ the one-plate-only line of recourse for your dinner course as well. Too many plates can make it challenging to keep track of portion size and can ultimately lead to overeating. To that end, stop eating directly from bags, packages, and cartons. Not only is it harder to measure how much you've eaten, but you may also fall victim to the, "I might as well just finish it," mindset and eat more just because it's there. Why is that a reason to eat more? Who cares if it's still there? Eat to satisfy your hunger—not because there are only a few pieces left, the expiration date is close, no one else wanted the item, or the refrigerator needs cleaning. Those aren't reasons. Finishing off that bag of chips may give you more space in your pantry, but there'll be less space in your pantsuit.

Post-Work Food Fest

It's also time to cut out the after-work binge that has become an occupational weight hazard for so many working people today. All too often, employees finish their workday absolutely famished to the point that they're racing through drive-throughs, ripping through their cupboards, and basically "eating a dinner before they eat dinner." But this type of modus operandi puts the pig in pig Latin and turns each night into an excessive eating experience. Plus, it's been shown that eating large dinners can make digestion more difficult and lead to weight gain. If you're repeatedly finding yourself stuffing your face uncontrollably after leaving work, it's time to reevaluate your afternoon and add a snack item into the routine. Since you're working up an appetite while at work, the trick is to have healthy afternoon foods available to you at your workplace and for your commute. That way, you don't have to arrive at home in the evening like a crazed beast ready to eat a horse. Staying ahead of your hunger throughout the day can enable and empower you to make rational and beneficial food choices that aren't guided by a grumbling stomach, but rather a thinking mind. Just like with any job assignment, you make the best decisions when you're levelheaded, clear-thinking, and in control, not when you're falling behind, frenetic, or frenzied. By preventing those frantic food feelings from ever occurring, you're setting the stage to place yourself and your weight loss goals first.

FINE DINING

"What's for dinner?" It's the inevitable question that comes toward the end of each workday. And yet, for so many intelligent working people, the answer ends up being a mystery wrapped in a calorific riddle. Instead of approaching dinner night after night like a chicken with your head cut off, it's time to assess your daily agenda and establish a plan that can eliminate the dinner guess-work caused by your job. The first step is to review your evening schedule and see which options make the most sense for you. Do you have time to prepare a meal upon returning home from work? If so, then the dinner world is your oyster, especially since there are numerous reasons why home cooking is a waist-saving solution. Not only can preparing a meal at home help save you dollars, it can also help save you pounds. This post-work strategy puts you in complete control over your dinner's contents, cost, cooking technique, and portion size. With this in mind, it's not surprising the word "chef" actually comes from the French word for "chief." You're the boss. You're the head honcho. So use your head and prepare a meal that benefits your body.

If You Cook

A simple online search can unlock countless healthy recipes and numerous light-inspired cookbooks filled with helpful options that can bring you closer to your weight loss goals. White fish with spinach. Rosemary chicken with green beans. Tofu stir-fry with peppers. There are also apps which can enable you to search through hundreds of beneficial recipes as well as filter by a certain ingredient or the total time you want to spend. Whether you have fifteen minutes or 150 minutes, there are lots of dinner options that can accommodate any time allotment. You can even find many apps that will do your grocery shopping for you, complete with delivery. Along these lines, a post-work technique is to apply your creativity to enlightening your go-to, tried-and-true recipes in every sense. You may know them by heart, but are they actually good for your heart? Now's the time to rewrite those signature dishes. One easy change is to examine your meals and look for simple swap outs. Trade in white rice for brown. Bake instead of fry. Choose quinoa over couscous. Try tomato sauce over cream. Serve kale chips instead of tortilla. Stop waiting to introduce food changes that benefit your body. Use this as an opportunity to try different recipes, experiment with new cooking tools, and incorporate unusual foods that you may not have tried. A related strategy is to sign up with one of the many companies that deliver recipes and all of the listed and measured ingredients you'll need to prepare a healthy dinner.

If You Don't Cook

If you're a person whose job makes it nearly impossible for you to prepare your own evening meal, you're not alone. It's the biting reality for countless individuals in countless industries. As a result, they've grown accustomed to fattening foodstuffs night after night—yes, grown. But regardless of the circumstances, even if you're short on time or long on excuses, you shouldn't let your work position put you in a foul food position. With a dash of forethought and a pinch of preparation, you can create an evening routine that doesn't involve a mad dash to find dinner—let alone a healthy dinner—in a pinch. Some post-work at-home dinner-reviving strategies include making and freezing healthy meals over the weekend so that they're ready to eat during the week. Utilizing prepackaged items and meal starter kits that can be spruced up with additions you already have in your pantry. Signing up for a service that delivers fresh and healthy dinners to your door. Consuming figure-friendly packaged frozen meals as well as heating up frozen vegetables as an easy side dish. Buying an additional healthy menu item while at lunch or finishing up your lunch leftovers. Purchasing a pre-cooked supermarket food such as a rotisserie chicken or making use of the salad bar. The bottom line is to eliminate the unknown dinner phenomenon which can inevitably lead to poor food choices.

RESTAURANT REALITIES

There are also the countless working individuals who've come to rely on outside eateries for their post-work dinner dining plans. Whether you're tired, lacking energy, want the cooking done for you, or are simply in the mood for something different, picking up a quick meal or going out to a restaurant is common practice in today's society, especially after a day on the job. In fact, there's a direct correlation between the amount of money spent on fast food and the number of hours worked. After all, when you're devoting more and more time to your job, the ease, speed, and convenience of these enticing eateries make them popular post-work choices day after day. More formal restaurants also have their appeal, of course, with delectable dishes, alluring ambiences, and exotic environments that can provide a nice change of pace from your office space. After dedicating hours upon hours to work, these opportunities to escape your corporate landscape are even more appealing. Not only do Americans spend almost half of their food budget on items they buy from foodservice providers such as fast food joints and restaurants, but it's a growing trend, with approximately $263 billion spent in 1992 and a whopping $415 billion spent in 2002. That's a 58 percent jump in ten years and a 23 percent increase when accounting for inflation. And speaking of inflation, this kind of eating behavior is further inflating the workforce.

Whether dining out or in, a problem with the food from many of these eateries is that portion sizes, calorie counts, and fat contents have gotten out of control in recent years. In fact, today's restaurant meals are nearly four times the size they were in the 1950s, with the average burger jumping from 3.9 ounces to twelve. Studies have consistently shown that a person tends to eat more sugar, salt, saturated fat, and around 200 extra calories when they dine out. Along these lines, a study in the *Journal of the American Dietetic Association* revealed that you're more likely to be overweight or obese when one or more dinners per week come from meals made outside of your home. Further, a University of Texas study found that dieting women ended up consuming around 225 to 250 extra calories and approximately ten to sixteen more grams of fat on days when they ate at restaurants—and these women were trying to lose weight!

MAKING DINNER WORK

The good news is that when you're eating an out-of-home dinner, there are strategies to prevent it from turning into a fat lot of good. Whether you're taking out or dining onsite, the first step is to gather as much information as possible about your food venue to help you determine the best post-work dinner strategy. Visit the eatery's website, search its menu, look at food photos, check out the calorie counts, and even read reviews. Collect as much data as possible regarding the food selections so that you can make a well-informed selection. Resolve ahead of time what you'll be consuming, no ifs, ands, or big butts. Craving Japanese food? Miso soup, steamed edamame, and veggie-filled sushi surpass fried tempura. Going Italian? Grilled chicken or fish outshines breaded veal. Choosing Chinese chow? Look for steamed meat and vegetables with sauces on the side instead of heavily smothered items such as sweet and sour pork. Also, toss the cookie and rewrite the fortune yourself—there's weight loss in your future.

Home-Course Advantage

For working people who pick up fast food or get takeout from a restaurant, make additions and subtractions to your meal with healthier items that you already have at home. Replace sandwich buns and breads with whole grain. Substitute your own oil-based salad dressing and supplement with your favorite veggies. Always ask for sauces and spreads on the side so that you can add your own lighter options as well as control their amount. It's up to you to make the necessary switches, swap outs, and substitutions when you're ordering. Another tip is to measure out the appropriate portion size of your meal when you arrive home and immediately put away the extra or split the meal with a family member. By doing so, you won't be tempted to overeat just because the food's in front of you. Out of sight, out of mouth. And speaking of temptation, ditch the dessert order. Not only does this save you some dough, but by the time you finish eating your meal, you may no longer be hungry for it. Plus, since research has shown that restaurant meals can be low on vitamins, eating fruits that you have on hand can make a great dessert option.

Shining While Dining Out

If your dinner plans involve dining at a restaurant, unleash your inner dining diva. Get the meal you want, the way you want. Period. It's called "ordering" after all. Not "suggesting." Not "hoping." Not "implying." But "ordering." Make the necessary changes and swap outs so that your dinner reflects your weight loss goals. Knowing what you're going to order before entering your dining destination is even more crucial in restaurants since they use every trick in the book to allure you with the sights, smells, and sounds of enticing eats, caloric concoctions, and fattening fare. It's also critical to avoid the common dining pitfalls that can take place when dining with others. If an appetizer is ordered for the table, you can place a small amount on your plate and eat directly from there. This will enable you to keep tabs on your portion size and help prevent overeating.

Speaking of appetizers, keep in mind that your main course doesn't have to come from the entrée section of the menu. This is where reviewing the restaurant's food photos can be helpful since you'll know ahead of time if an appetizer is size S or size XXXXXL. To that end, since portion sizes at dining destinations tend to be larger than life, share a meal with a co-diner or request that the meal be divided in the kitchen and set aside for you to take home. You're not missing out on tonight's dinner but gaining tomorrow's lunch. And in terms of gaining, forethought and planning are particularly important when it comes to dessert, as deciding ahead of time lets you adjust the size and content of your main course as well as helps you fight off temptation. If dessert is ordered for the table to share, you can always separate out a taste for yourself if you truly want it. But keep your weight goals in mind. If a simple dollop of dessert will turn your cravings into overdrive, then pump the brakes. It's so not worth it. But you are.

SO MUCH FOR YOUR SIX PACK

For many people, having a drink is a popular way to unwind after a hectic workday. Whether out on the town or in the comfort of their own home, employees often choose to incorporate booze into their evening. In some cases, coworkers decide to hit up a happy hour at a local bar, pub, or even fancy hotel lounge and enjoy some drinks and snacks after work. It's a fun way to socialize, kick back, and have some laughs after a day on the job, but if you're not careful, you can end up packing on the pounds after pounding beers with your colleagues. Alcohol is loaded with calories, and it actually contains more calories per gram than both carbohydrates and protein. And when considering the common foodstuffs available at happy hours today, it's no wonder that getting tipsy can tip the scales. With offerings like chili cheese fries, pork nachos, and fried mozzarella sticks, happy hours can result in many unhappy hours of regret.

Bars also use a plethora of techniques to entice you to order more and more, such as serving complimentary pretzels, nuts, and other salty snacks. Since your body uses water to rid itself of the sodium found in these foods, you're bound to feel thirsty and crave another drink or two. Plus, research has shown that people tend to drink faster and drink more when loud music is playing in the bar. And happy hours lure you in with reduced pricing during certain hours, further incentivizing bar-goers to order more food and drinks. This gives new meaning to the expression, penny-wise, pound-foolish.

How to Handle Happy Hours

Fortunately, when it comes to work happy hours, there are steps that can keep you and your weight in good spirits. First, as is the case when visiting any type of food location, look online and do the appropriate due diligence regarding the venue of choice. Find out everything you can in terms of its offerings, foodstuff selection, and drink types so you can establish a plan before entering. To that end, predetermine a drink maximum for yourself—such as one to two drinks—especially since slight intoxication around coworkers can be problematic. You may end up saying or doing something extraordinarily foolish. With this in mind, it's important to predetermine what type of drink(s) you plan on ordering, especially since alcoholic beverages can be calorific nightmares. Do you really need a mudslide for 610 calories? Or a mai tai for 406 calories? Or a piña colada for 366 calories? Sure, the tiny umbrella in the drink is cute, but the rains will soon follow. Instead of downing drinks that double as desserts, one popular choice of savvy drinkers whether you're out on the town or not is red wine. At only 120 calories, studies have shown drinking red wine in moderation can be a heart-healthy choice and has been linked to lowering LDL cholesterol in the blood. In fact, the antioxidants in wine have been shown to help prevent blood clots and blood vessel damage, and may also help improve memory. If that's not memorable enough, a study from Purdue University revealed that another compound in red wine can help block the processes that enable the formation of fat cells. If that's not a big, fat "cell-ing" point for red wine, then what is?

If red wine still doesn't do it for you, there are plenty of other drink options that raise the bar. And that's not just sour grapes. If you're a beer fan, lighter beer options are the way to go as they typically have less carbs than regular beer but contain the same alcohol content. Other drinking tips include ditching the sweet and sugary mixers found in so many specialty cocktails and ordering a flavor-infused vodka on the rocks to save calories. It's also a good idea to opt for body-friendly mixers such as diet soda, club soda, diet tonic, and juices such as lemon, lime, grapefruit, and low-cal cranberry or orange. If you're more of a cocktail connoisseur, some lower-calorie cocktails that won't make a mockery of your weight goals include a bloody Mary (118 calories), an apple martini (148 calories), and a mojito (212 calories). You also shouldn't hesitate to bust out the bubbly, especially since champagne has only 110 calories. It may not be New Year's Eve, but taking control of your weight is definitely worth celebrating.

When it comes to happy-hour eating, preparing ahead of time can prevent your own bar food fight. One strategy is to eat an afternoon snack since it'll make you less likely to engorge on happy hour crap simply because you're hungry after work.

It's also vital to plan on having dinner after your happy hour. All too often, working people attend happy hours without thinking about their dinner plans, and they frequently find themselves overindulging on fatty food just because it's in front of them. By refraining from treating happy hour foodstuffs as though they're your main meal, you'll feel less inclined to stuff your face.

Another tip of happy happy-hour-goers is to only order food items with your first drink order. As the drinks keep flowing, it's too easy to be tempted to keep ordering more and more as your inebriation level grows and grows. Plan on ordering when you arrive, and that's it. And just as in any other food venue, don't hesitate to make healthy changes to the items you order such as requesting mini sliders without the buns so you can minimize your own buns.

You should also take the initiative to locate happy hour spots that serve healthier options. Venues that serve hummus platters or tomato mozzarella skewers do exist if you make the effort to find them. To that end, when the bar food arrives, no matter what it is, separate out a portion for yourself onto your own plate and eat directly from there. Don't go back for seconds, thirds, or tenths. This enables you to keep track of your portion size, prevents overeating, and can even help slow down the pace of your eating and drinking since you already have the full amount you plan on ingesting right in front of you. Also, try to avoid consuming the complimentary pretzels and nuts that the bar provides. Not only is it hard to keep track of the gross total that you ate, but it's actually just totally gross. How long have these snacks been sitting out? Whose hands were in there before yours? These free snacks are worth just as much to your body as what you paid for them.

OVERTIME AND OVERWEIGHT

Whether you're hourly or salaried, trading in time at home for time at the office is simply part of the trade. If you're putting in extra hours night after night, you're not alone. Staying late to wrap up reports, finalize presentations, and complete assignments has become commonplace in the workplace. In fact, Americans work more hours on average than employees in most other industrialized countries. Even Silicon Valley has its own lingo regarding the extra work hours that companies expect their staff to put in during certain parts of the year. For those in the software development industry, "crunch time" is known as the time period in which employees work additional hours to finish projects, fix bugs, and make various modifications to meet a looming deadline. But these supplemental hours can really add up. In fact, a survey of over 1,000 game developers revealed that during a typical crunch time, 69 percent work fifty-one to eighty hours per week—or more! And this can last for a few months. It's not surprising that those surveyed also reported crunch time's detrimental impact on their well-being. Shouldn't that be the bug that needs fixing?

Behind the Extra Hours

There are several reasons why people today are working longer hours. One main factor is that there's simply too much work for employees to handle during the workday. Also, in light of widespread downsizing, a greater workload has been falling on fewer employees, and as a result they need more time to do their jobs. In addition, late-night hours are often required when communicating with clients and colleagues in different time zones or overseas. Plus, extra hours provide an opportunity for workers to get ahead on demanding assignments and projects, and some employees even enjoy the less-hectic after-hours office setting in order to get their work done. For hourly employees, an additional incentive is the increased hourly rate—time and a half—for such work. Employees can also feel pressured to stay late on the job because they don't want to appear unmotivated, unchallenged, or uncommitted, especially if their manager is still at the office. While you might feel or hope that the extra hours you're working are worth it, this is definitely worth a second look. It's been found that some nations with the highest amount of hours worked per employee actually have close to the lowest levels of productivity. More specifically, productivity is not correlated with hours worked, and it can be argued that it's actually more disadvantageous. Long hours can take their toll on a worker's creativity, efficiency, and outlook, and it's been shown that working overtime is also associated with a lower performance on neuropsychological tests. With this in mind, burning the midnight oil can often lead to employee burnout.

It's clear that excessive hours can take a toll on your health. As published in the *International Journal of Obesity*, a study of nearly 9,000 Helsinki city employees revealed that working overtime and work exhaustion are associated with weight gain. Even the CDC warns about the potential pitfalls of working overtime, as it's been linked to a higher frequency of illnesses, lower assessment of health, increased probability of injuries, greater likelihood of smoking or alcohol use, and of course, increases in weight. It's almost as if working overtime should come with its own warning label, although this may be a hard pill to swallow. The problem is that many employees spend these long hours filling themselves with fattening foodstuffs disguised as fuel. In a word, crunch time easily becomes munch time. Overtime puts you at risk for consuming extra calories that you wouldn't necessarily be taking in if you weren't working, and it's likely those added calories will be stored as fat.

OVERTIME OVERHAUL

Fortunately, you can revamp your long hours so that they don't leave you long in the waistband. A go-to strategy is to set a plan for what you'll be eating during these hours. All too often, employees make crappy overtime food choices due to a lack of time, forethought, and preparation. They distractedly down sugary snacks, chomp on chips while churning out reports, and eat one dinner at 7:00 p.m. and another one at 10:00 p.m. While you may return home with your work completed, you're completely food defeated. But by planning ahead to make healthy options available during the extra hours, you and your work will come out ahead. One effective option is to bring a dinner from home in anticipation of working extended hours, and in such a case, you could also heat up a frozen meal or purchase an extra meal during lunch. In terms of food choices, you can also take a tip from night shift workers and consume foods that are high in protein such as fish, white meat chicken, and white meat turkey, all of which are energy boosters.

Order of Operations

If your p.m. routine is usually to order in with colleagues, stop working for a second, scour the restaurant's online menu for a minute, and take the moments you need to nail down the choices that best align with your weight loss goals. A stitch in time saves nine pounds. And speaking of ordering, a common late-night staple delivered to so many offices today is pizza. It's quick, convenient, and can appease crowds of coworkers both small and large. The good news is that eating pizza without turning from small to large isn't just a pizza pie in the sky. To counter pizza poundage, a hot tip is to spice it up. Studies have shown that capsaicin, a compound found in red chili pepper, can help boost your metabolism and help burn more calories. Additionally, eating spicy foods may also increase your feelings of fullness and decrease your appetite. If that doesn't get you fired up, another pizza approach is to order a thin crust—or a whole grain crust—and ask for half of the usual amount of cheese or pull off some of the cheese yourself. By doing so, you can save on calories, carbs, and saturated fat since pizza is one of the top sources of saturated fat in the American diet.

It's also important to get saucy. Lycopene, a carotenoid that gives tomatoes their red color, is not only an antioxidant that can help protect cells from free radicals and may aid in reducing the risk of certain cancers, research has also shown that increased levels of lycopene in the blood are tied to a lower risk of stroke. In a word, the right pizza isn't white pizza. In terms of toppings, load your slice with veggies and replace processed meats like pepperoni with leaner proteins like chicken. And be sure to put your pizza under the knife, as supersized slices can cut your weight loss journey short. A very palatable strategy is to first place only one piece of pizza onto your plate and divide that piece in half. This approach can cut both ways, as it's possible you won't even need to go back to the box for the "second slice" since you'll technically be eating two slices. Another pizza proposition is to turn your sides into starters. Many pizza parlors serve salads, and research from Pennsylvania State University revealed that women who ate large salads filled with carrots, tomatoes, cucumbers, celery, and a low-fat dressing prior to their main meal consumed approximately 100 less total calories than at meals where they didn't eat salad. That's exciting news no matter how you slice it.

The Buzz on Caffeine

Excess hours often cause employees to down excess caffeine—coffee concoctions, sweetened sodas, and energy beverages—to power through their excessive workload. Aside from the added sugar, calories, and potentially dangerous side effects of so-called energy-inducing drinks, too much caffeine has been linked to copious health issues, including obesity. Keep in mind that the recommended safe amount of caffeine per day is 400 mg, which is roughly equal to four cups of brewed coffee. As many night shift workers know, there are ways to stay energized without chugging caffeinated drinks, such as walking around, taking a brief nap, listening to pump-up music, staying hydrated, and conversing with coworkers. If you do decide to suck down caffeine, ingest it toward the beginning of your extra hours since having it later in the evening may make it more difficult to fall asleep that night. And that would suck.

EXERCISE THE DEMONS

Finding the time, energy, and motivation to work out after work can be tough work. You've been on the job all day, and sometimes the idea of having to fit in a workout so you can fit into a smaller size may leave you fit to be tied. While slacking off doesn't cut it in your work-life, employees may find themselves slacking off in their workout-life, which often results in less slack in their slacks. But exercise is a crucial component of any successful and lasting weight management program, and it needs to be made a priority. The first step is to predetermine a set time to exercise during the evening so that you can plan each night accordingly. Block out your workout times on your calendar, just as you do for meetings and tasks at work. Since you're conditioned to keep your appointments on job matters, it'll be that much easier for you to respond in the same way to matters that deal with your physical conditioning.

Right after Work

One popular evening exercise strategy is to work out directly after work. By adhering to this type of schedule, you're laying the groundwork to turn exercising into a habitual routine. Research has continued to demonstrate the powerful impact that habits and rituals have on goal attainment. As noted in the *Journal of Personality and Social Psychology*, people are more likely to cling to habits, both good and bad, when they're tired or under stress. By working to instill new habits that benefit your weight, you're more likely to continue these behaviors even when faced with outside pressures from your job. To that end, researchers contend that developing new and favorable habits can even be more powerful than merely trying to apply self-control and willpower. Additionally, consuming the right foods at the right time before your after-work workout can further help lock in your exercise habit so you're not tempted to blow off the gym because of hunger. Eating a snack such as a banana with a spoonful of peanut butter, yogurt and blueberries, or a low-fat granola bar approximately forty-five minutes prior to exercising, along with staying hydrated, can help empower you during your workout while simultaneously fighting feelings of hunger and sluggishness.

Fitting Attire

Another go-to strategy for busy employees engaging in a post-work workout is to change into their exercise clothes before leaving the office. By doing so, you'll be less likely to pass right by the gym, Pilates studio, or spinning class after leaving work since you've already swapped your business suit for a track suit. And speaking of exercise clothes, an additional motivational move is to invest in workout gear that you actually enjoy wearing. Replace your ratty running shoes with a pair that's comfortable and supportive. Get rid of your socks with holes for a whole new set of socks. Trade in your torn shirt for a style, color, and cut that you want to put on so you can take the pounds off. When you're feeling confident about what you're wearing, you're often more inclined to challenge yourself during your workout and less inclined to skip it. Plus, many sport retailers offer complimentary local exercise clubs and classes.

Through Thick and Thin

An additional technique that can ramp up your post-work workout motivation is to buddy up. As reported in the *Archives of Internal Medicine*, research has found that people who exercise with a companion tend to lose more weight. Not only do you and your workout partner inspire, impel, and incentivize each other to push harder during your workout, but the buddy system can also help boost your exercise commitment and consistency by holding you accountable to another person or persons. Plus, it can make your workout more enjoyable. Why not gather a group of coworkers and spend time together at the gym after work? Ask your cubicle neighbors to accompany you for a post-work walk around your business's neighborhood. You can also conduct workout sessions without even having to leave your office. Not only can these exercise opportunities improve your physical strength, but they also strengthen camaraderie, collaboration, and cooperation.

Friends with Benefits

Keep in mind that the buddy method isn't just for you and your coworkers, as you can always invite others to accompany you on your exercise expedition. Rather than meeting a friend at a bar before dinner, meet her at a barre workout session. Take advantage of apps that offer discounted exercise classes and head with a pal to a Pilates studio. There are also websites that help you find post-work exercise groups in your area as well as online programs that can enable you to register for different workout classes and studios across the United States. And while it may be difficult to work up a conversation while you're working up a sweat, dinner is next on the agenda. To that end, use your recent workout as inspiration and motivation to engage in healthy dinner dining habits. Why undo the good you just did? Would you ever delete a great report that you just finished writing?

After Dinner Movements

Another option for busy working people is to work out after dinner. Exercise studios offer late-night sessions, many gyms are open 24/7, and getting into a yoga child's pose position can be a nice reward after helping your child with his homework. The trick for late-night exercisers is to find a workout time and type that's conducive to your evening schedule. In terms of timing, some say to wait at least two hours after your meal before strenuous exercise in order to digest your dinner and prevent cramps and feelings of sluggishness. But don't dismay if you can't wait that long. In fact, research has shown that walking approximately fifteen minutes after eating not only burns calories, but can also assist in both digestion and blood sugar control. As discussed in a study published in the *Journal of the American Medical Directors Association*, individuals with type 2 diabetes who walked for twenty minutes shortly after dinner helped lower their blood sugar more effectively than those who walked before dinner. Even more clearly, a small study has shown that walking within an hour of your meal can be an effective strategy for weight loss. By experimenting with different exercise regimens within the parameters of your evening, you can find a workout type and time that complement your schedule and your body.

Excuses, Excuses

There are many working people who avoid regular late-night workout sessions because they believe it'll inhibit their sleeping. It's time to put this misconception to rest. Sleep researchers contend that while there may be a small group of individuals who experience some sort of sleep delay, most people don't have any sleep issues when exercising close to their bedtime. In fact, a study in the *Journal of Sleep Research* found that late-night exercise isn't a factor in the disturbance of sleep, as individuals experienced the same sleep quality on nights when they exercised right before bed as well as on nights when they didn't. Plus, according to the 2013 National Sleep Foundation's "Sleep in America Poll," the vast majority of individuals who exercised—no matter what time of day—reported that they had a better night's sleep than individuals who didn't exercise at all. No more excuses.

THE REST IS HISTORY

For large numbers of working people in today's workforce, getting enough sleep happens once in a blue moon. It's often recommended that adults sleep between seven to nine hours per night, and yet a 2013 Gallup Poll revealed that 40 percent of Americans sleep six hours or less per night. One of the main causes behind this stirring phenomenon is that your job is preventing you from getting a good night's rest, and this ugly truth is costing you more than just your beauty sleep. With the growing trend in longer work hours, when nightfall comes people often find themselves spending time on their work matters instead of on their mattress. In fact, 40 percent of American employees are still checking their office emails after 10:00 p.m., and with 70 percent of workers considering this to be an essential step before bed, it's clear that your job trumps your jammies. The reality for workers today is that a pushed-up deadline inevitably means a pushed-back bedtime. And when you finally do manage to get to bed, your work has crawled right in with you, since extreme demands, difficult bosses, and pressure-laden presentations can keep your mind buzzing with office buzz long into the night. Too many working people end up counting job stressors each night instead of counting sheep.

Technological Awakenings

The technology employed by employees to keep them connected to their jobs is also at fault for keeping them up. Not only are many workers held responsible for responding to late-night job issues such as a text from a manager, an overseas email from a client, or a frantic phone call from a coworker, but the devices themselves are literally contributing to your sleep drought. A study from the Lighting Research Center (LRC) at Rensselaer Polytechnic Institute revealed that staring at the short-wavelength light emitted by electronic devices like smartphones and tablets before bed can cause your body to slow or suppress the production of melatonin, the hormone which regulates your body's sleep cycle. This can contribute to a poorer night's sleep by reducing sleep onset as well as sleep duration. And when considering the increasing sizes of these devices as well as the proximity that people tend to hold them in relation to their face, each new product launch is generating more and more unrest.

Sleeping and Weighty Issues

As working people lose more and more sleep, they end up gaining more and more weight. A study from the Perelman School of Medicine at the University of Pennsylvania revealed that the later you go to bed and the less sleep you get, the more likely you are to gain weight. In fact, not only are you more prone to eat before bed during these late-night hours, researchers also determined that the types of food and drink consumed in these later hours tended to be higher in fat and calories than those consumed during earlier times throughout the day. Further, through the use of brain scans, a study conducted at the University of

California, Berkeley, determined that a sleepless night can impair your ability to make complex decisions while also stimulating the part of your brain associated with seeking rewards. Consequently, participants craved high-fat and high-sugar foods when they were sleep deprived as opposed to when they were rested. Even more telling, a study published in the *American Journal of Epidemiology* which followed over 60,000 women for sixteen years determined that those who slept for five hours or less each night had a 15 percent greater likelihood of becoming obese than women who had seven hours of sleep each night. In a word, it's clear that depriving yourself of sleep is setting the stage for future weight gain.

Less Sleep, More Problems

If the increased poundage due to sleep loss isn't a big enough nightmare for you, a lack of sleep is also linked to a smorgasbord of other serious problems. Specifically, sleep deprivation is associated with an increased risk of heart disease, type 2 diabetes, high blood pressure, stroke, mental illness, substance dependency, and even premature death. If you're neglecting sleep because your work philosophy is, "You'll sleep when you're dead," this may end up being a self-fulfilling prophecy. A lack of sleep can also be hard on your sex drive and has been linked to fertility impairment. Individuals who are chronically sleep deprived may also experience an earlier onset of dementia and Alzheimer's disease, as was determined by Temple University researchers using a mouse model. To that end, as published in the *Journal of Neuroscience*, a separate study on mice revealed that sleep deprivation can damage a certain kind of brain cell which plays a role in your ability to stay up and alert. Keep that in mind the next time you're neglecting sleep because you're caught up in your job's rat race.

Work Woes as Sleep Goes

Sleep deprivation isn't just harming your body, it's also harming your work. Not only are you more likely to make mistakes, have accidents, forget things, and employ poorer judgment when working without adequate sleep, but staying up late to get ahead is actually putting you behind. Harvard researchers determined that employee sleep deprivation is costing American companies an estimated $63.2 billion per year in lost productivity. Face it, how many times have you found it difficult to concentrate at work because you've felt a bit drowsy? Or perhaps you've sensed your eyes getting heavy during a midday meeting? There can be many instances when your lack of sleep negatively impacts your job performance and output, but the problems don't end there. A study published in the *Journal of Occupational Health Psychology* revealed that sleeping for less than six hours per night is the main risk factor for developing on-the-job burnout. In essence, being tired from your job can inevitably make you tired of your job.

SHUT-EYE STRATEGIES

The good news is that there are numerous ways to prevent your job from stifling your weight loss dreams. Sleep has to be made a priority, and that responsibility falls on you. One step is to keep a spreadsheet documenting your time spent in bed. Whether you're doing this manually or using various apps available today, it's imperative to establish a benchmark regarding your bedtime, sleep quantity, and even sleep quality. Once you have a clearer picture of your sleep patterns, you can begin to implement positive changes and adjustments. Your goal should be to create a weekly bed schedule—the bed sched—and follow it as you follow important schedules at work. If you want to be in bed by 10:00 p.m., do everything in your power to get your butt in bed by 10:00 p.m. Additionally, by going to bed and waking up around the same time each day, you're helping regulate your body's internal clock as well as aiding your sleeping abilities, daily energy levels, and weight loss.

When Duty Calls

Once you've documented your actual rest regimen, you're in a much better position to identify and deal with the possible sources of your sleep shortage. Are you up at night because you're doing work for your job? If so, one option is to reexamine your workday and determine if there are any missed opportunities to employ more effective time management, delegation, or assertiveness. Perhaps your manager is unaware that he's overloading you with work—he's likely to continue to do so until you speak up. Be open and businesslike and don't hesitate to stand up for yourself and your health. Communication can play a major role in ending sleep deprivation. To that end, another sleep-saving step is to limit your nightly work-related availability within reason. Perhaps your constant responsiveness to late-night calls, emails, and texts has indicated to others that it's okay to contact you at any hour. Stop rewarding the very behavior that you're trying to extinguish. Refute this repute and notify colleagues that you're not going to be accessible after a specific time unless there's an emergency.

Restfulness, Not Restlessness

If you typically get restless when you're trying to rest, rest assured—a good night's sleep doesn't have to be a pipe dream. Many working individuals end up tossing and turning at night because they're having a hard time turning off their racing mind. Whether you're feeling anxious about an upcoming meeting or are simply unsure of what to wear to work the next day, your thoughts may still be zipping even when you want to catch some zzzs. If you're finding it challenging to shut it off when you shut your eyes, the trick is to write down everything that's on your mind. Getting your thoughts and feelings out can enable you to better manage what's speeding through your head and can help you get a fresh perspective. In addition, the act of physically writing out your thoughts can help make whatever's on your mind more tangible, controllable, and easier to manage. To that end, another tactic that can facilitate your desire to rest a bit easier is to check out the vast array of sleep-assisting resources available today. Using earplugs, blackout curtains, and eye masks can give you that extra edge to edge out sleeplessness, and you can also take advantage of noise machine apps. If you prefer falling asleep to the sound of raindrops, the ocean, or simply white noise, you can find the idyllic backdrop to take back sleep and drop weight.

Sleeping Potpourri

Other strategies for a good night's sleep include ingesting sleep-friendly foods and beverages for dinner or as a low-calorie nighttime snack. Consuming foodstuffs such as warm milk, nuts, and whole grains can help facilitate sleep. Plus, stop chugging late-night beverages that are loaded with caffeine and kiss them all goodnight. You should also really think before you have a late-night drink, as booze can impair your ability to snooze. Additionally, investing in new pajamas, new pillows, or even a new mattress can help. If you still feel unable to fall asleep throughout the night, remaining in bed is your best bed bet. You can do some deep breathing or even light meditation while lying in the dark. Don't get angry, don't get up, and don't give up. Create the opportunity for sleep success so that you can have weight loss success—that's the sweetest dream of all.

Epilogue

Food for Thought
and Thoughts for Food

While there's no question that your job is making you fat, there's also no question that you can now focus your knowledge, skills, drive, perseverance, and goal orientation to counter this counterproductive force.

LOOKING TO THE FUTURE

When you approach a serious, high-level, and long-term assignment, you do so with considerable up-front planning and organizing, accompanied by detailed monitoring and course corrections along the way—all in an effort to successfully meet the objectives. It wouldn't make any business sense whatsoever to simply wing it on a project, weighty or not. With proven tools, techniques, and strategies at your fingertips, you now have just what you need to reach your weight loss goals. But as is the case with your job responsibilities, nothing happens until you step up and drive the process.

A WORK IN PROGRESS

As is the case with any major project, you may encounter some turbulence along the way. Perhaps you felt that you ate too many cookies at a coworker's birthday party, so you decided to flip into engorgement mode and stuff your face with fatty foods for the rest of the day. Eliminate this black and white thinking that allows you to sabotage yourself because you believe that you had one slip-up. After all, if you feel you made an error on a project, you wouldn't then deliberately undermine the rest of your work going forward. Rather, when you make a mistake on an assignment, you deal with it, you learn from it, and you move on. This is the same methodology you should apply when you encounter a bump on your weight loss journey.

YOU'RE IN CHARGE

Whether you're in management or not, you're actually a manager—you're the manager of yourself. And just like a corporation, you have several departments to oversee. You organize your finances. You advertise and market your abilities. You sell your labor. You provide goods and services. You do long-term planning. You invest in growth and development. But there's one additional area directly under your leadership that needs major attention—your infrastructure. In fact, the word "corporation" comes from the Latin "corpus" which means "body." Failing to effectively manage your body opens the door to powerful job-related factors that can weigh it down to the point of collapse. Fortunately, you have the power to take clear, specific, measurable, and businesslike actions to overcome the hefty hostile takeover attempts lodged against you each workday. What are you waiting for?

Acknowledgments

I n a nutshell, we would like to give special shout-outs to some of the people whose support for this project literally brought it to fruition. Thanks to Joelle Delbourgo and her team at Joelle Delbourgo Associates, as well as Krishan Trotman, Diane Wood, and the staff at Skyhorse Publishing.

Thanks also to Ken's workplace advice column readers and to those who highlighted concerns about food-related issues on their jobs. And to Jessica Lloyd, MD, Perrin F. Disner, Attorney at Law, and Professor Sandy Jacoby, thanks for being such helpful resources. And finally, to our family, thanks for your insights, inspiration, and inordinate patience as this book about weight loss consumed much of our time.

Bibliography

"A Little Fat Helps the Vegetables Go Down." *WebMD* 27 July 2004. 15 Jan. 2015. <http://www.webmd.com/food-recipes/news/20040727/fat-helps-vegetables-go-down>.

"A workout at work?" *The Washington Post* 6 Sept. 2011. 20 Jan. 2015. <http://www.washingtonpost.com/wp-srv/special/health/workout-at-work/>.

"About The Blood Alcohol Concentration Estimate." *HealthStatus* 17 Jan. 2015. <http://www.healthstatus.com/calculate/blood-alcohol-bac-calculator>.

Albertson, Ann M., Sandra G. Affenito, and Nandan Joshi. "Ready-to-Eat Cereal Consumption Patterns and the Association with Body Mass Index and Nutrient Intake in American Adults." *Journal of Nutrition and Food Sciences* 2.5 (2002). 14 Jan. 2015. <http://omicsonline.org/ready-to-eat-cereal-consumption-patterns-and-the-association-with-body-mass-index-and-nutrient-intake-in-american-adults-2155-9600.1000145.pdf>.

"Alcohol Awareness." *Police Department: The University of Georgia* 4 Dec. 2014. 16 Jan. 2015. <http://www.police.uga.edu/alcoholawareness.html>.

"Alcohol, Nutrition, & Healthy Eating." *Washington State University ADCAPS* 18 Jan. 2015. <http://adcaps.wsu.edu/alcohol101/alcohol,-nutrition,-healthy-eating/>.

American Cancer Society. "Eating at fast food, full service restaurants linked to more calories, poorer nutrition." *ScienceDaily* 7 August 2014. 18 Jan. 2015. <http://www.sciencedaily.com/releases/2014/08/140807105211.htm>.

American Chemical Society. "Drink water to curb weight gain? Clinical trial confirms effectiveness of simple appetite control method." *ScienceDaily* 23 Aug. 2010. 17 Jan. 2105. <www.sciencedaily.com/releases/2010/08/100823142929.htm>.

American Psychological Association. "Telecommuting has mostly positive consequences for employees and employers." *ScienceDaily* 20 November 2007.

16 Jan. 2015. <www.sciencedaily.com/releases/2007/11/071119182930. htm>.

Ansel, Karen. "Packing the Perfect Cooler." *Home Food Safety* 15 Jan. 2015. <http://homefoodsafety.org/refrigerate/packing-cooler>.

Anwar, Yasmin. "Sleep deprivation linked to junk food cravings." *UC Berkeley News Center* 6 Aug. 2013. 18 Jan. 2015. <http://newscenter.berkeley. edu/2013/08/06/poor-sleep-junk-food/>.

Arble, Deanna M., et al. "Circadian timing of food intake contributes to weight gain." *Obesity (Silver Spring)* 17.11 (2009): 2100-2102. PubMed. gov. 17 Jan. 2015. <http://www.ncbi.nlm.nih.gov/pubmed/19730426>.

Aschwanden, Christie. "Deskbound? Here's how much you need to stand or move to stay healthy." *The Washington Post* 20 July 2015. <http://www.wash-ingtonpost.com/national/health-science/deskbound-heres-how-much-you-need-to-stand-or-move-to-stay-healthy/2015/07/20/7ab35878-2a59-11e5-bd33-395c05608059_story.html>.

Associated Press. "Exercise balls as office furniture." *NBCNews.com* 7 Nov. 2012. 24 Jan. 2015. <http://www.nbcnews.com/id/3404446/ns/ health-fitness/t/exercise-balls-office-furniture/#.VMR74nsrmlc>.

Au, N., K. Hauck, and B. Hollingsworth. "Employment, work hours and weight gain among middle-aged women," *International Journal of Obesity* 37 (2013): 718-724. Nature.com. 12 Jan. 2015. <http://www.nature. com/ijo/journal/v37/n5/full/ijo201292a.html>.

Baikie, Karen A., and Kay Wilhelm. "Emotional and physical health benefits of expressive writing." *Advances in Psychiatric Treatment* 11 (2005): 338-346. 22 Jan. 2015. <http://apt.rcpsych.org/content/11/5/338.full>.

Barton, J., J. Aldridge, and P. Smith. "Emotional impact of shift work on the children of shift workers." *Scandinavian Journal of Work, Environment & Health* 24.3 (1998): 146-150. 17 Jan. 2015. <http://www.sjweh. fi/show_abstract.php?abstract_id=350>.

Ben-Ner, Avner, et al. "Treadmill Workstations: The Effects of Walking while Working on Physical Activity and Work Performance." *PLoS One* 20 Feb. 2014. 20 Jan. 2015. <http://journals.plos.org/plosone/arti-cle?id=10.1371/journal.pone.0088620>.

"Benefit of drinking green tea: The proof is in – drinking tea is healthy, says Harvard Women's Health Watch." *Harvard Health Publications: Harvard*

Medical School Sept. 2004. 14 Jan. 2015. <http://www.health.harvard.edu/press_releases/benefit_of_drinking_green_tea>.

Booth, Stephanie. "How to choose the best frozen dinners." *WebMD* 31 July 2014. 17 Jan. 2015. <http://www.webmd.com/diet/features/best-frozen-dinners>.

Boston, Gabriella. "Fruit juice has benefits, but calories outweigh them, experts say." *The Washington Post* 16 Oct. 2012. 14 Jan. 2015. <http://www.washingtonpost.com/lifestyle/wellness/fruit-juice-has-benefits-but-calories-outweigh-them-experts-say/2012/10/15/6809bb2e-f2c9-11e1-adc6-87dfa8eff430_story.html>. Bouchez, Colette. "Can Stress Cause Weight Gain?" *WebMD* 13 May 2005. 21 Jan. 2015. <http://www.webmd.com/diet/features/can-stress-cause-weight-gain>.

Bouchez, Colette. "Choosing a Weight Loss Buddy." *WebMD* 9 Feb. 2011. 23 Jan. 2015. <http://www.webmd.com/diet/features/choosing-weight-loss-buddy>.

Bouchez, Colette. "Exercise for Energy: Workouts That Work." *WebMD* 7 Aug. 2009. 22 Jan. 2015. <http://www.webmd.com/fitness-exercise/features/exercise-for-energy-workouts-that-work>.

Bradt, J., C. Dileo, and M. Shim. "Music interventions for preoperative anxiety." *Cochrane Database of Systematic Reviews* 6:CD0069086 (2013). PubMed.gov. 17 Jan. 2015. <http://www.ncbi.nlm.nih.gov/pubmed/23740695>.

Brandt, Michelle. "Pedometers help people stay active, Stanford study finds." *Stanford Medicine News Center* 20 Nov. 2007. 23 Jan. 2015. <http://med.stanford.edu/news/all-news/2007/11/pedometers-help-people-stay-active-stanford-study-finds.html>.

"Breakfast is key for health says research." *University of Bath* 13 Jan. 2015. <http://www.bath.ac.uk/research/news/2014/06/05/bath-breakfast-study/>.

Bresiger, Gregory. "Millions of Americans skipping lunch to work: study." *New York Post* 2 Feb. 2014. 15 Jan. 2015. <http://nypost.com/2014/02/02/millions-of-americans-skipping-lunch-to-work-study/>.

Bridger, Haley. "You are when you eat: Study may help explain increased risk of diabetes in shift workers." *Harvard Gazette* 13 Apr. 2015. <http://news.harvard.edu/gazette/story/2015/04/you-are-when-you-eat/>.

British Psychological Society (BPS). "Office workers spend too much time at their desks, experts say." *ScienceDaily* 15 Jan. 2012. 18 Jan. 2015. <http://www.sciencedaily.com/releases/2012/01/120113210203.htm>.

Buman, Matthew P., et al. "Does nighttime exercise really disturb sleep? Results from the 2013 National Sleep Foundation Sleep in America Poll." *Sleep Medicine* 15.7 (2014): 755-761. 19 Jan. 2015. <http://www.sleep-journal.com/article/S1389-9457(14)00045-8/abstract>.

Cahill, Leah E., et al. "Prospective Study of Breakfast Eating and Incident of Coronary Heart Disease in a Cohort of Male US Health Professionals." *Circulation* 128 (2003): 313-314. 13 Jan. 2015. <http://circ.ahajournals.org/content/128/4/337.abstract>.

Carls, G.S., et al. "The impact of weight gain or loss on health care costs for employees at the Johnson & Johnson Family of Companies. *Journal of Occupational and Environmental Medicine / American College of Occupational and Environmental Medicine* 53.1 (2011): 8-16. PubMed.gov. 20 Jan. 2015. <http://www.ncbi.nlm.nih.gov/pubmed/21187786>.

Caruso, Claire C., et al. "Overtime and Extended Work Shifts: Recent Findings on Illnesses, Injuries, and Health Behaviors." *Centers for Disease Control and Prevention: Workplace Safety and Health* April 2004. U.S. Department of Health and Human Services. 18 Jan. 2015. <http://www.cdc.gov/niosh/docs/2004-143/pdfs/2004-143.pdf>.

Cassidy, Aedín, et al. "High Anthocyanin Intake Is Associated With a Reduced Risk of Myocardial Infarction in Young and Middle-Aged Women." *Circulation* 127 (2013): 188-196. 14 Jan. 2015. <http://circ.ahajournals.org/content/127/2/188.full>.

Castillo, Michelle. "You are what your peers eat: Study shows others' eating habits affect individual choices." *CBS News* 2 Jan. 2014. 15 Jan. 2015. <http://www.cbsnews.com/news/you-are-what-your-peers-eat-study-shows-societal-consumption-affects-individual-choices/>.

CBSNews. "How Americans Eat Today." *CBS News* 12 Jan. 2010. 18 Jan. 2015. <http://www.cbsnews.com/news/how-americans-eat-today/>.

Cell Press. "How a protein meal tells your brain you're full." *Science Daily* 5 July 2012. 17 Jan. 2015. <www.sciencedaily.com/releases/2012/07/120705172041.htm>.

Chan, Amanda L. "6 Reasons To Not Go Out To Dinner Tonight." *HuffPost: The Third Metric* 19 Aug. 2014. 18 Jan. 2015. <http://www.huffington-post.com/2014/08/16/eating-out-calories-health-_n_5660010.html>.

Christian, T.J. "Trade-offs between commuting time and health-related activities." *Journal of Urban Health* 89.5 (2012): 746-757. PubMed.gov. 17 Jan. 2015. <http://www.ncbi.nlm.nih.gov/pubmed/22689293.1>.

Christian, Thomas James. "Opportunity Costs Surrounding Exercise and Dietary Behaviors: Quantifying Trade-offs Between Commuting Time and Health-Related Activities." *Social Science Research Network* 28 Apr. 2013. 17 Jan. 2015. <http://papers.ssrn.com/sol3/papers.cfm?abstract_id=1490117>.

Church, Timothy S., et al. "Trends over 5 Decades in U.S. Occupation-Related Physical Activity and Their Associations with Obesity." *PLoS One* 25 May 2011. 12 Jan. 2015. <http://www.plosone.org/article/info%3Adoi%2F10.1371%2Fjournal.pone.0019657>.

Clarke, Janine, and Ian Janssen. "Is the frequency of weekly moderate-to-vigorous physical activity associated with the metabolic syndrome in Canadian adults?" *Applied Physiology, Nutrition, and Metabolism* 38.7 (2013). 14 Jan. 2015. <http://www.nrcresearchpress.com/doi/abs/10.1139/apnm-2013-0049#.VLcklZUtHIU>.

"Coffee Health Risks: For the moderate drinker, coffee is safe says Harvard Women's Health Watch." *Harvard Health Publications: Harvard Medical School* Aug. 2004. 14 Jan. 2015. <http://www.health.harvard.edu/press_releases/coffee_health_risk>.

Cohen, Jennifer. "9 Bad Habits That Make You Fat." *Forbes* 24 Apr. 2012. 15 Jan. 2015. <http://www.forbes.com/sites/jennifercohen/2012/04/24/9-bad-habits-that-make-you-fat/>.

Colberg, S.R., et al. "Postprandial walking is better for lowering the glycemic effect of dinner than pre-dinner exercise in type 2 diabetic individuals." *Journal of the American Medical Directors Association* 10.6 (2009): 394-397. PubMed.gov. 18 Jan. 2015. <http://www.ncbi.nlm.nih.gov/pubmed/19560716>.

Collingwood, Jane. "The Physical Effects of Long-Term Stress." *PsychCentral* 21 Jan. 2015. <http://psychcentral.com/lib/the-physical-effects-of-long-term-stress/000935>.

Collins, Karen. "The Salad Strategy to Control Weight." *American Institute for Cancer Research* 31 July 2006. 18 Jan. 2015. <http://preventcancer.aicr.org/site/News2?page=NewsArticle&id=10038&news_iv_ctrl=0&abbr=pr_hf_>.

"Common Signs & Signals of a Stress Reaction." *Federal Occupational Health* U.S. Department of Health and Human Services. 23 Jan. 2015. <http://www.foh.dhhs.gov/NYCU/StressReaction.asp>.

Creswell, J. David, et al. "Self-Affirmation Improves Problem-Solving under Stress." *PLoS One* 1 May 2013. 23 Jan. 2015. <http://journals.plos.org/plosone/article?id=10.1371/journal.pone.0062593>.

Dahl, Melissa. "Science of Us: At Work, Every Friday Should Be a Summer Friday." *NYMag* 29 Aug. 2014. 18 Jan. 2015. <http://nymag.com/scienceofus/2014/08/work-every-friday-should-be-a-summer-friday.html>.

Dallas, Mary Elizabeth. "Too Much Sitting Linked to Chronic Health Problems." *WebMD* 21 Feb. 2013. 17 Jan. 2015. <http://www.webmd.com/heart-disease/news/20130221/too-much-sitting-linked-to-chronic-health-problems>.

"Desktop Dining Survey: 2011 Results Americans' Food Safety Knowledge and Practice at Work." *Home Food Safety* Apr. 2011. 15 Jan. 2015. <http://homefoodsafety.org/vault/2499/web/files/Desktop%20Dining%20Executive%20Summary%20FINAL.pdf>.

DiChiara, Tom. "Can exercising at night hurt your sleep?" *CNN* 22 Apr. 2014. 19 Jan. 2015. <http://www.cnn.com/2014/04/22/health/upwave-night-exercise/>.

Doheny, Kathleen. "Fatigue Fighters: 6 Quick Ways to Boost Energy." *WebMD* 19 Nov. 2010. 17 Jan. 2015. <http://www.webmd.com/diet/fiber-health-benefits-11/fatigue-fighters-six-quick-ways-boost-energy?page=1>.

Doheny, Kathleen. "Sitting Too Much: How Bad Is It?" *WebMD* 7 April 2014. 19 Jan. 2015. <http://www.webmd.com/fitness-exercise/news/20140407/sitting-disease-faq>.

"Doing Good Is Good for You: 2013 Health and Volunteering Study." *United-Health Group* 2013. 23 Jan. 2015. <http://www.unitedhealthgroup.com/~/media/UHG/PDF/2013/UNH-Health-Volunteering-Study.ashx>.

"Don't Fall Prey to Portion Distortion." *American Heart Association* 9 Jan. 2015. 18 Jan. 2015. <http://www.heart.org/HEARTORG/Getting-

Healthy/WeightManagement/LosingWeight/Dont-Fall-Prey-to-Portion-Distortion_UCM_424567_Article.jsp>.

Downs, Martin. "Healthy 'Briefcase Breakfasts'" *WebMD* 17 Mar. 2006. 14 Jan. 2015. <http://www.webmd.com/food-recipes/features/healthy-briefcase-breakfasts>.

Dugan, Andrew. "Fast Food Still Major Part of U.S. Diet." *Gallup* 6 Aug. 2013. 18 Jan. 2015. <http://www.gallup.com/poll/163868/fast-food-major-part-diet.aspx>.

Dunham, Will. "Weight of the world: 2.1 billion people obese or over-weight." *Reuters* 28 May 2014. 12 Jan. 2015. <http://www.reuters.com/article/2014/05/28/us-health-obesity-idUSKBN0E82HX20140528>.

Durston, James. "Airline 'fat tax': Should heavy passengers pay more?" *CNN: International* 26 Mar. 2013. 16 Jan. 2015. <http://travel.cnn.com/airline-fat-tax-should-heavy-passengers-pay-more-619046>.

"Eat Well @ Work." *University Health Services Tang Center @ Berkeley* 15 Jan. 2015. <http://www.uhs.berkeley.edu/facstaff/healthmatters/eatwel-latwork.shtml>.

"Eating low-fat yogurt may help prevent Type 2 diabetes: study." *Daily News* 7 Feb. 2014. 14 Jan. 2015. <http://www.nydailynews.com/life-style/health/eating-low-fat-yogurt-prevent-type-2-diabetes-study-article-1.1606387>.

Eberly, Robin, and Harvey Feldman. "Obesity and Shift Work in the General Population." *The Internet Journal of Allied Health Sciences and Practices* 8.3 (2010). 17 Jan. 2015. <http://ijahsp.nova.edu/articles/Vol8Num3/pdf/feldman.pdf >.

Edgar, Julie. "Types of Teas and Their Health Benefits." *WebMD* 20 March 2009. 14 Jan. 2015. <http://www.webmd.com/diet/features/tea-types-and-their-health-benefits>.

"Email 'vacations' decrease stress, increase concentration." *UC Health* 3 May 2012. 22 Jan. 2015. <http://health.universityofcalifornia.edu/2012/05/03/email-vacations-decrease-stress-increase-concentration/>.

Evans, Lisa. "Why You Should Let Your Employees Nap at Work." *Entrepreneur* 24 Aug. 2014. 22 Jan. 2015. <http://www.entrepreneur.com/article/236755>.

"Factoids—What you always wanted to know about alcohol and drugs." *Washington State University ADCAPS* 18 Jan. 2015. <http://adcaps.wsu.edu/factoids/>.

"FAST FOOD: Survey Reveals Lunch Break for Nearly Half of Workers Is 30 Minutes or Less; Most Spend That Time Socializing With Colleagues." *OfficeTeam: A Robert Half Company* 16 Jan. 2014. 15 Jan. 2015. <http://officeteam.rhi.mediaroom.com/lunchbreaks>.

"FastStats: Obesity and Overweight." *Centers for Disease Control and Prevention* 7 Jan. 2015. 12 Jan. 2015. <http://www.cdc.gov/nchs/fastats/obesity-overweight.htm>.

Fernandez, Diana. "Rochester Study Connects Workplace Turmoil, Stress and Obesity." *University of Rochester Medical Center* 24 Mar. 2010. 21 Jan. 2015. <http://www.urmc.rochester.edu/news/story/index.cfm?id=2803>.

Fernandez, Isabel Diana, et al. "Association of Workplace Chronic and Acute Stressors With Employee Weight Status: Data From Worksites in Turmoil." *Journal of Occupational and Environmental Medicine* 52.1S (2010): S34-S41. 20 Jan. 2015. <http://journals.lww.com/joem/Abstract/2010/01001/Association_of_Workplace_Chronic_and_Acute.7.aspx>.

Finkelstein, Eric A., et al. "The Costs of Obesity in the Workplace." *Journal of Occupational and Environmental Medicine* 52.10 (2010): 971-976. 20 Jan. 2015. <http://journals.lww.com/joem/Abstract/2010/10000/The_Costs_of_Obesity_in_the_Workplace.4.aspx>.

Fisher, Anne. "Your job might be killing you." *Fortune* 2 Apr. 2013. 21 Jan. 2015. <http://fortune.com/2013/04/02/your-job-might-be-killing-you/>.

Flint, Ellen, Steven Cummins, and Amanda Sacker. "Associations between active commuting, body fat, and body mass index: population based, cross sectional study in the United Kingdom." *The BMJ* 349:g4887 (2014). 17 Jan. 2015. <http://www.bmj.com/content/349/bmj.g4887>.

"Food Safety Information: How Temperatures Affect Food." *United States Department of Agriculture Food Safety and Inspection Service* May 2011. 15 Jan. 2015. <http://www.fsis.usda.gov/shared/PDF/How_Temperatures_Affect_Food.pdf>.

Fox, Emily Jane. "Work from home soars 41% in 10 years." *CNN: Money* 4 Oct. 2012. 16 Jan. 2015. <http://money.cnn.com/2012/10/04/news/economy/work-from-home/index.html>.

Fox, Justin. "Instinct Can Beat Analytical Thinking." *Harvard Business Review* 20 June 2014. 17 Jan. 2015. <https://hbr.org/2014/06/instinct-can-beat-analytical-thinking>.

Fryer, Bronwyn. "Sleep Deficit: The Performance Killer." *Harvard Business Review* Oct. 2006. 17 Jan. 2015. <https://hbr.org/2006/10/sleep-deficit-the-performance-killer>.

Fryer, Shari. "News & Events: Just One-In-Five Employees Take An Actual Lunch Break." *Right Management: ManPowerGroup* 16 Oct. 2012. 15 Jan. 2015. <http://www.right.com/news-and-events/press-releases/2012-press-releases/item23943.aspx>.

Fulkerson, J.A., et al. "Away-from-home family dinner sources and associations with weight status, body composition, and related biomarkers of chronic disease among adolescents and their parents." *Journal of the American Dietetic Association* 111.12 (2011): 1892-1897. PubMed.gov. 18 Jan. 2015. <http://www.ncbi.nlm.nih.gov/pubmed/22117665>.

Geiger, Sylvia M. "You can fit restaurant fare into a healthy lifestyle." *Chicago Tribune* 9 May 2012. 18 Jan. 2015. <http://articles.chicagotribune.com /2012-05-09/lifestyle/sns-201205081600—tms—premhnstr—k-h20120509 may09_1_restaurant-industry-food-restaurants-restaurant-meals>.

"Get up! New research shows standing meetings improve creativity and teamwork." *Washington University in St. Louis* 12 June 2014. 19 January 2015. <http://news.wustl.edu/news/Pages/27031.aspx>.

Gifford, Julia. "Here's Proof That Standing Desks Make You More Productive." *Business Insider* 27 Sept. 2013. 20 Jan. 2015. <http://www.businessinsider.com/proof-standing-desks-you-more-productive-2013-9>.

Godman, Heidi. "Lycopene-rich tomatoes linked to lower stroke risk." *Harvard Health Publications: Harvard Medical School* 10 Oct. 2012. 18 Jan. 2015. <http://www.health.harvard.edu/blog/lycopene-rich-tomatoes-linked-to-lower-stroke-risk-201210105400>.

Goldberg, Joseph. "Depression Health Center: Exercise and Depression." *WebMD* 19 Feb. 2014. 17 Jan. 2015. <http://www.webmd.com/depression/guide/exercise-depression>.

Goldsmith, Belinda. "Third of Office Workers Skip Breakfast: Survey." *Reuters* 23 Nov. 2007. 5 Jan. 2015. <http://in.reuters.com/article/2007/11/23/us-food-breakfast-idINN2331826220071123>.

González, R., et al. "Effects of flavonoids and other polyphenols on inflammation." *Critical Reviews in Food Science and Nutrition* 51.4 (2011): 331-362. PubMed.gov. 14 Jan. 2015. <http://www.ncbi.nlm.nih.gov/pubmed/21432698>.

Granados, K., et al. "Appetite regulation in response to sitting and energy imbalance." *Applied Physiology, Nutrition, and Metabolism* 37.2 (2012): 323-333. PubMed.gov. 18 Jan. 2015. <http://www.ncbi.nlm.nih.gov/pubmed/22462636>.

Graves, Jada A., and Katy Marquardt. "The Vanishing Lunch Break." *U.S. News & World Report: Money* 9 Oct. 2013. 15 Jan. 2015. <http://money.usnews.com/money/careers/articles/2013/10/09/the-vanishing-lunch-break-2>.

Gregoire, Carolyn. "Yoga Associated With Gene Expression In Immune Cells, Study Finds." *HuffPost: Healthy Living* 30 Apr. 2013. 23 Jan. 2015. <http://www.huffingtonpost.com/2013/04/24/yoga-immune-system-genetic-_n_3141008.html>.

Gurian, Anita. "Family meals matter—staying connected." *The Child Study Center: NYU Langone Medical Center* 18 Jan. 2015. <http://www.aboutourkids.org/articles/family_meals_matter—staying_connected>.

Hallett, Vicky, and Lenny Bernstein. "Even if you can't bike or walk to work, you can get exercise while commuting." *The Washington Post* 7 Oct. 2010. 17 Jan. 2015. <http://www.washingtonpost.com/wp-dyn/content/article/2010/10/05/AR2010100502128.html>.

Han, Kihye, et al. "Comparison of Job Stress and Obesity in Nurses With Favorable and Unfavorable Work Schedules." *Journal of Occupational and Environmental Health Medicine* 54.8 (2012): 928-932. <http://journals.lww.com/joem/Abstract/2012/08000/Comparison_of_Job_Stress_and_Obesity_in_Nurses.5.aspx>.

Hansson, Erik, et al. "Relationship between commuting and health outcomes in a cross-sectional population survey in southern Sweden." *BMC Public Health* 834.11 (2011). 17 Jan. 2015. <http://www.biomedcentral.com/1471-2458/11/834/abstract>.

Hatfield, Heather. "7 Tips for Eating While You Work." *WebMD* 12 Dec. 2008. 15 Jan. 2015. <http://www.webmd.com/food-recipes/features/7-tips-eating-while-you-work>.

Hayashi, Alden M. "When to Trust Your Gut." *Harvard Business Review* Feb. 2001. 20 Jan. 2015. <https://hbr.org/2001/02/when-to-trust-your-gut/ar/1>.

"Healthy Nuts: Health Benefits For Almonds, Walnuts, Cashews, Peanuts And More." *HuffPost: Healthy Living* 6 May 2013. 17 Jan. 2015. <http://www.huffingtonpost.com/2013/05/06/healthy-nuts-health-benefits-cashews-walnuts-peanuts-almonds_n_3187731.html>.

"Healthy Weight—it's not a diet, it's a lifestyle!" *Centers for Disease Control and Prevention* 13 Sept. 2011. 17 Jan. 2015. <http://www.cdc.gov/healthyweight/losing_weight/eating_habits.html>.

Healy, Melissa. "Study says: Financial reward + competition = More weight loss." *Los Angeles Times* 1 Apr. 2013. 23 Jan. 2015. <http://articles.latimes.com/2013/apr/01/news/la-heb-weight-loss-group-money-20130401>.

Hellmich, Nanci. "Q&A: How to drop pounds with all-day activities, not exercise." *USA Today* 22 Jan. 2009. 18 Jan. 2015. <http://usatoday30.usatoday.com/news/health/weightloss/2009-01-21-fidget-activity_N.htm>.

Hendriksen, I.J., et al. "The association between commuter cycling and sickness absence." *Preventive Medicine* 51.2 (2010): 132-5. PubMed.gov. 17 Jan. 2015. <http://www.ncbi.nlm.nih.gov/pubmed/20580736>.

Hevrdejs, Judy. "Desks: Dirtier than Toilet Seats." *Chicago Tribune* 5 Sept. 2011. 15 Jan. 2015. <http://articles.chicagotribune.com/2011-09-05/features/ct-tribu-lunch-hour-dirty-desks-20110905_1_desks-toilet-seat-bacteria>.

Hijikata, Yasuyo, and Seika Yamada. "Walking just after a meal seems to be more effective for weight loss than waiting for one hour to walk after a meal." *International Journal of General Medicine* 4 (2011): 447-450. PMC. 18 Jan. 2015. <http://www.ncbi.nlm.nih.gov/pmc/articles/PMC3119587/>.

Hinter, Geraldine. "Work stress triggers road rage." *University of South Australia* 7 Sept. 2009. 21 Jan. 2015. <http://w3.unisa.edu.au/unisanews/2005/february/workstress.asp>.

Hitti, Miranda. "Do Work Woes Bring Weight Gain?" *WebMD* 17 May 2005. 18 Jan. 2015. <http://www.webmd.com/diet/news/20050517/do-work-woes-bring-weight-gain>.

Hitti, Miranda. "Heartier Benefits Seen from Oatmeal." *WebMD* 11 Jan. 2008. 14 Jan. 2015. <http://www.webmd.com/cholesterol-management/news/20080111/heartier-benefits-seen-from-oatmeal>.

Hitti, Miranda. "Pedometers Motivate Weight Loss." *WebMD* 14 Jan. 2008. 23 Jan. 2015. <http://www.webmd.com/fitness-exercise/news/20080114/pedometers-motivate-weight-loss>.

Hitti, Miranda. "Traffic Stress? Cinnamon, Peppermint May Help." *WebMD* 28 Apr. 2005. 17 Jan. 2015. <http://www.webmd.com/food-recipes/news/20050428/traffic-stress-cinnamon-peppermint-may-help>.

Hobson, Katherine. "6 Ways to Make Working The Night Shift Less Hazardous to Your Health." *U.S. News & World Report: Health* 4 Dec. 2009. 17 Jan. 2015. <http://health.usnews.com/health-news/family-health/sleep/articles/2009/12/04/6-ways-to-make-working-the-night-shift-less-hazardous-to-your-health>.

Holmes, Lindsay. "9 Things Only People With Depression Can Truly Understand." *HuffPost: Stronger Together* 26 Aug. 2014. 17 Jan. 2015. <http://www.huffingtonpost.com/2014/08/26/depression-frustrations_n_5692649.html>.

"How much physical activity do adults need?" *Centers for Disease Control and Prevention* 3 Mar. 2014. 23 Jan. 2015. <http://www.cdc.gov/physicalactivity/everyone/guidelines/adults.html>.

Hsu, Tiffany. "Average Americans work a day of overtime each week." *Los Angeles Times* 3 July 2012. 13 Jan. 2015. <http://articles.latimes.com/2012/jul/03/business/la-fi-mo-overtime-20120703>.

Hyman, Mark. "10 Reasons to Quit Your Coffee!" *HuffPost: Healthy Living* 31 Oct. 2012. 14 Jan. 2015. <http://www.huffingtonpost.com/dr-mark-hyman/quit-coffee_b_1598108.html>.

"Insufficient Sleep Is A Public Health Epidemic." *Centers for Disease Control and Prevention* 13 Jan. 2014. 18 Jan. 2015. <http://www.cdc.gov/features/dssleep/>.

Jacobs, Emily. "The healthiest and unhealthiest breakfast foods." *Fox News* 25 June 2014. 15 Jan. 2015. <http://www.foxnews.com/leisure/2014/06/25/healthiest-and-unhealthiest-breakfast-foods/>.

Jacques, Renee. "9 Unfortunate Truths about Juicy, Scrumptious Bacon." *HuffPost: Taste* 14 Nov. 2013. 13 Jan. 2015. <http://www.huffingtonpost.com/2013/11/12/bacon-facts_n_4241592.html>.

Johnson, Alison. "How to order a healthy pizza." *Chicago Tribune* 7 Mar. 2010. 19 Jan. 2015. <http://articles.chicagotribune.com/2010-03-07/health/sc-health-0303-howto-pizza-20100303_1_thin-crust-feta-cheese-pizza>.

Jones, Jeffery M. "In U.S., 40% Get Less Than Recommended Amount of Sleep." *Gallup* 19 Dec. 2013. 18 Jan. 2015. <http://www.gallup.com/poll/166553/less-recommended-amount-sleep.aspx>.

Kadlec, Dan. "How To Save $2,500 a Year on Lunch." *Time* 29 Aug. 2012. 15 Jan. 2015. <http://business.time.com/2012/08/29/how-to-save-2500-a-year-on-lunch/>.

Kaplan, Karen. "Does milk do a body good? Maybe not, a new study suggests." *Los Angeles Times* 29 Oct. 2014. 14 Jan. 2015. <http://www.latimes.com/science/la-sci-sn-milk-health-risks-20141029-story.html#page=1>.

Kaplan, Karen. "Obese Americans now outnumber those who are merely overweight, study says." *Los Angeles Times* 22 June 2015. <http://www.latimes.com/science/la-sci-sn-more-americans-obese-than-over-weight-20150620-story.html>.

Kapp, Diana. "Does It Count as a Family Dinner If It's Over in Eight Minutes?" *The Wall Street Journal* 17 Sept. 2013. 18 Jan. 2015. <http://www.wsj.com/articles/SB10001424127887323981304579079720375700820>.

Kessler, Ronald C., et al. "Insomnia and the Performance of US Workers: Results from the America Insomnia Survey." *Sleep* 34.9 (2011): 1161-1171. PMC. 19 Jan. 2015. <http://www.ncbi.nlm.nih.gov/pmc/articles/PMC3157657/>.

Kirkpatrick, Kristin. "5 Foods That Help You Sleep." *HealthHub from Cleveland Clinic* 12 June 2014. 19 Jan. 2015. <http://health.clevelandclinic.org/2014/06/5-foods-that-help-you-sleep/>.

Komaroff, Anthony. "Study supports heart benefits from Mediterranean-style diets." *Harvard Health Publications* 25 Feb. 2013. 23 Jan. 2015. <http://www.health.harvard.edu/blog/study-supports-heart-benefits-from-mediterranean-style-diets-201302255930>.

Kulinski, Jaquelyn P., et al. "Association Between Cardiorespiratory Fitness and Accelerometer-Derived Physical Activity and Sedentary Time in the General Population." *Mayo Clinic Proceedings* 89.8 (2014): 1063-1071. 24 Jan. 2015. <http://www.mayoclinicproceedings.org/article/S0025-6196%2814%2900382-6/abstract>.

Lallukka, T., et al. "Psychosocial working conditions and weight gain among employees." *International Journal of Obesity (London)* 29.8 (2005): 909-915. PubMed.gov. 18 Jan. 2015. <http://www.ncbi.nlm.nih.gov/pubmed/15852046>.

"Late Bedtimes Lead to Larger Waistlines, Penn Medicine Study Finds." *Penn Medicine: News Brief* 28 June 2013. 18 Jan. 2015. <http://www.uphs.upenn.edu/news/News_Releases/2013/06/spaeth/>.

Lawrence, Jean. "Exercise at Your Desk." *WebMD* 27 Feb. 2004. 19 Jan. 2015. <http://www.webmd.com/fitness-exercise/features/exercise-at-your-desk>.

Lemaire, Jane B., et al. "Food for thought: an exploratory study of how physicians experience poor workplace nutrition." *Nutrition Journal* 10 (2011). PMC. 15 Jan. 2015. <http://www.ncbi.nlm.nih.gov/pmc/articles/PMC3068081/?tool=pubmed>.

"Less processed meat, more fish and exercise may boost sperm count, quality." *Harvard T.H. Chan School of Public Health* 2013. 13 Jan. 2015. <http://www.hsph.harvard.edu/news/hsph-in-the-news/less-processed-meat-more-fish-and-exercise-may-boost-sperm-count-quality/>.

Levine, J.A., S.J. Schleusner, and M.D. Jensen. "Energy expenditure of non-exercise activity." *The American Journal of Clinical Nutrition* 72.6 (2000): 1451-1454. PubMed.gov. 19 Jan. 2015. <http://www.ncbi.nlm.nih.gov/pubmed/11101470>.

Levine, James. "Killer Chairs: How Desk Jobs Ruin Your Health." *Scientific American* 311.5 (2014). 20 Jan. 2015. <http://www.scientificamerican.com/article/killer-chairs-how-desk-jobs-ruin-your-health/>.

Levine, James. "What are the risks of sitting too much?" *Mayo Clinic* 16 June 2012. 20 January 2015. <http://www.mayoclinic.org/healthy-living/adult-health/expert-answers/sitting/faq-20058005>.

Lewis, Tanya. "Health: Red wine compound may improve memory, study suggests." *Fox News* 9 June 2014. 18 Jan. 2015. <http://www.foxnews.

com/health/2014/06/09/red-wine-compound-may-improve-memory-study-suggests/>.

"Light weights are just as good for building muscle, getting stronger, researchers find." *McMaster University* 30 April 2012. 20 Jan. 2015. <http://www.mcmaster.ca/opr/html/opr/media/main/NewsReleases/Lightweightsare-justasgoodforbuildingmusclegettingstrongerresearchersfind.htm>.

Linn, Allison. "More Companies Look To Hire Employees Who Aren't Jerks." *HuffPost: Business* 5 Oct. 2013. 22 Jan. 2015. <http://www.huffingtonpost.com/2013/10/05/companies-hire-jerks_n_4045336.html>.

Lloyd, Ken. *151 Quick Ideas to Recognize and Reward Employees.* Franklin Lakes: The Career Press, 2007.

"Low Pay, Commute Top Reasons 80% of Americans Stressed at Work." *Corinthian Colleges, Inc.* 9 Apr. 2014. 17 Jan. 2015. <http://newsroom.cci.edu/releasedetail.cfm?ReleaseID=839103>.

Lourida, I., et al. "Mediterranean diet, cognitive function, and dementia: a systematic review." *Epidemiology* 24.4 (2013): 479-489. PubMed.gov. 24 Jan. 2015. <http://www.ncbi.nlm.nih.gov/pubmed/23680940>.

Luckerson, Victor. "Is Lunch a Waste of Time—Or a Productivity Booster?" *Time* 16 July 2012. 15 Jan. 2015. <http://business.time.com/2012/07/16/the-lunch-hour-necessity-or-nuisance/>.

Ma, Yunsheng, et al. "Association Between Eating Patterns And Obesity In A Free-living US Adult Population." *American Journal of Epidemiology* 158.1 (2003): 85-92. Oxford Journals. 5 Jan. 2015. <http://aje.oxford-journals.org/content/158/1/85.full#sec-5>.

MacDonald, Ann. "Harvard Health Blog: Why eating slowly may help you feel full faster." *Harvard Health Publications: Harvard Medical School* 19 Oct. 2010. 15 Jan. 2015. <http://www.health.harvard.edu/blog/why-eating-slowly-may-help-you-feel-full-faster-20101019605>.

MacMillan, Amanda. "Top 20 Foods to Eat for Breakfast." *ABC News* 1 June 2013. 14 Jan. 2015. <http://abcnews.go.com/Health/Wellness/top-20-foods-eat-breakfast/story?id=19295525#>.

Macrae, Fiona. "Why sitting still is the best way to work up an appetite." *Daily Mail* 25 Sept. 2008. 19 Jan. 2015. <http://www.dailymail.co.uk/health/article-1061462/Why-sitting-best-way-work-appetite.html#ixzz3LHvJVlu6 >.

Magee, Christopher A., et al. "Occupational Factors Associated With 4-Year Weight Gain in Australian Adults." *Journal of Occupational and Environmental Medicine* 52.10 (2010): 977-981.20 Jan. 2015. <http://journals.lww.com/joem/Abstract/2010/10000/Occupational_Factors_Associated_With_4_Year_Weight.5.aspx>.

Magee, Elaine. "Healthy Breakfast Ideas and Recipes." *WebMD* 3 Apr. 2008. 14 Jan. 2015. <http://www.webmd.com/food-recipes/features/healthy-breakfast-ideas-and-recipes>.

Magee, Elaine. "The Benefits of Yogurt." *WebMD* 7 Mar. 2007. 15 Jan. 2015. <http://www.webmd.com/diet/features/benefits-of-yogurt>.

Magee, Elaine. "The Best Bread: Tips for Buying Breads." *WebMD* 2009. 14 Jan. 2015. <http://www.webmd.com/food-recipes/features/the_best_bread_tips_for_buying_breads>.

Magee, Elaine. "The Best of the Bars." *WebMD* 26 July 2005. 14 Jan. 2015. <http://www.webmd.com/diet/features/the-best-of-the-bars>.

Mann, Denise. "Coping With Excessive Sleepiness: Can Better Sleep Mean Catching Fewer Colds?" *WebMD* 19 Jan. 2010. 17 Jan. 2015. <http://www.webmd.com/sleep-disorders/excessive-sleepiness-10/immune-system-lack-of-sleep>.

Mann, Denise. "The Sleep-Diabetes Connection." *WebMD* 19 Jan. 2010. 19 Jan. 2015. <http://www.webmd.com/sleep-disorders/excessive-sleepiness-10/diabetes-lack-of-sleep?page=2>.

Mann, Denise. "Trans Fats: The Science and the Risks." *WebMD* 6 July 2006. 12 Jan. 2015. <http://www.webmd.com/diet/features/trans-fats-science-and-risks>.

Marksberry, Kellie. "Take a Deep Breath." *The American Institute of Stress* 10 Aug. 2012. 17 Jan. 2015. <http://www.stress.org/take-a-deep-breath/>.

Matthews, C.E., et al. "Amount of time spent in sedentary behaviors and cause-specific mortality in US adults." *The American Journal of Clinical Nutrition* 95.2 (2012): 437-445. PubMed.gov. 20 Jan. 2015. <http://www.ncbi.nlm.nih.gov/pubmed/22218159>.

Max-Planck-Gesellschaft. "Pictures of food create feelings of hunger." *ScienceDaily* 19 Jan. 2012. 17 Jan. 2015. <www.sciencedaily.com/releases/2012/01/120119101713.htm>.

Maxon, Rebecca. "Stress in the Workplace: A Costly Epidemic." *FDU Magazine: Fairleigh Dickinson University* Summer 1999. 22 Jan. 2015. <http://www.fdu.edu/newspubs/magazine/99su/stress.html>.

Mayo Clinic Staff. "Chronic stress puts your health at risk." *Mayo Clinic* 11 July 2013. 21 Jan. 2015. <http://www.mayoclinic.org/healthy-living/stress-management/in-depth/stress/art-20046037>.

Mayo Clinic Staff. "Diseases and Conditions: Dehydration." *Mayo Clinic* 12 Feb. 2014. 16 Jan. 2015. <http://www.mayoclinic.org/diseases-conditions/dehydration/basics/definition/con-20030056>.

Mayo Clinic Staff. "Eating and exercise: 5 tips to maximize your workouts." *Mayo Clinic* 21 Feb. 2014. 15 Jan. 2015. <http://www.mayoclinic.org/healthy-living/fitness/in-depth/exercise/art-20045506?pg=1>.

Mayo Clinic Staff. "Exercise and stress: Get moving to manage stress." *Mayo Clinic* 21 July 2012. 22 Jan. 2015. <http://www.mayoclinic.org/healthy-living/stress-management/in-depth/exercise-and-stress/art-20044469>.

Mayo Clinic Staff. "Meditation: A simple, fast way to reduce stress." *Mayo Clinic* 19 July 2014. 22 Jan. 2015. <http://www.mayoclinic.org/tests-procedures/meditation/in-depth/meditation/art-20045858?pg=1>.

Mayo Clinic Staff. "Office exercise: Add more activity to your workday." *Mayo Clinic* 8 Feb. 2014. 20 January 2015. <http://www.mayoclinic.org/healthy-living/adult-health/in-depth/office-exercise/art-20047394?pg=1>.

Mayo Clinic Staff. "Red wine and resveratrol: Good for your heart?" *Mayo Clinic* 25 Apr. 2015. 18 Jan. 2015. <http://www.mayoclinic.org/diseases-conditions/heart-disease/in-depth/red-wine/art-20048281>.

Mayo Clinic Staff. "Stress symptoms: Effects on your body and behavior." *Mayo Clinic* 19 July 2013. 21 Jan 2015. <http://www.mayoclinic.org/healthy-living/stress-management/in-depth/stress-symptoms/art-20050987?pg=1>.

Mayo Clinic Staff. "Walking: Make it count with activity trackers." *Mayo Clinic* 21 Feb. 2014. 23 Jan. 2015. <http://www.mayoclinic.org/healthy-living/fitness/in-depth/walking/art-20047880?pg=1>.

Mayo Clinic Staff. "Yoga: Fight stress and find serenity." *Mayo Clinic* 15 Jan. 2013. 22 Jan. 2015. <http://www.mayoclinic.org/healthy-living/stress-management/in-depth/yoga/art-20044733>.

McDonnell, Amy K. "Let Them Eat Cake: Why Workers Are Gaining Weight." *The Hiring Site Blog powered by CareerBuilder* 6 June 2012. 12 Jan. 2015. <http://thehiringsite.careerbuilder.com/2012/06/06/american-workers-are-gaining-weight/>.

McKenzie, Brian, and Melanie Rapino. "Commuting in the United States: 2009." *U.S. Department of Commerce* Sept. 2011. 17 Jan. 2015. <http://www.census.gov/prod/2011pubs/acs-15.pdf>.

"Medicines in my Home: Caffeine and Your Body." *U.S. Food and Drug Administration* 2007. 17 Jan. 2015. <http://www.fda.gov/downloads/drugs/resourcesforyou/consumers/buyingusingmedicinesafely/understandingover-the-countermedicines/ucm205286.pdf>.

"Mediterranean Diet Associated with Longer Telomeres." *Brigham and Women's Hospital* 2 Dec. 2014. 23 Jan. 2015. <http://www.brighamandwomens.org/about_bwh/publicaffairs/news/pressreleases/PressRelease.aspx?PageId=1943>.

Mekary, Rania A., et al. "Eating patterns and type 2 diabetes risk in older women: breakfast consumption and eating frequency." *The American Journal of Clinical Nutrition* 12 June 2013. 13 Jan. 2015. <http://ajcn.nutrition.org/content/early/2013/06/12/ajcn.112.057521.abstract>.

Mendez, Barbara. "7 Foods That Reduce Stress." *Inc.* 17 June 2013. 17 Jan. 2015. <http://www.inc.com/barbara-mendez/7-foods-that-reduce-stress.html>.

Messing, Laurie. "Parent's Influence Children's Eating Habits: Be a good role model for your kids by eating healthy." *Michigan State University Extension* 3 April 2013. 13 Jan. 2015. <http://msue.anr.msu.edu/news/parents_influence_childrens_eating_habits>.

Miller, Kelli. "Skip Breakfast, Get Fat." *WebMD* 15 June 2009. 13 Jan. 2015. <http://www.webmd.com/diet/news/20090615/skip-breakfast-get-fat>.

Miller, Patrick, and Brad Bulkley. "Game Developer Quality-of-Life Survey." *Gamasutra: The Art & Business of Making Games* 18 March 2013. 18 Jan. 2015. <http://www.gamasutra.com/view/feature/188671/game_developer_qualityoflife_.php>.

Mills, Harry, et al. "Visualization and Guided Imagery Techniques for Stress Reduction." *MentalHelp.net* 30 June 2008. 23 Jan. 2015. <http://www.mentalhelp.net/poc/view_doc.php?type=doc&id=15672>.

Moisse, Katie. "Commuting to Work Linked to Health Problems." *ABC News* 31 Oct. 2011. 16 Jan. 2015. <http://abcnews.go.com/Health/Wellness/commuting-work-linked-health-worries/story?id=14846412>.

Moisse, Katie. "Sugar Dubbed Dangerous, Addictive Drug." *ABC News* 18 Sept. 2013. 12 Jan. 2015. <http://abcnews.go.com/blogs/health/2013/09/18/sugar-dubbed-dangerous-addictive-drug>.

Moninger, Jeannette. "10 Relaxation Techniques That Zap Stress Fast." *WebMD* 30 Sept. 2013. 22 Jan. 2015. <http://www.webmd.com/balance/guide/blissing-out-10-relaxation-techniques-reduce-stress-spot>.

Moretz, Preston. "Chronic sleep disturbance might trigger onset of Alzheimer's." *Temple University Health Center* 18 Mar. 2014. 18 Jan. 2015. <http://news.temple.edu/news/2014-03-18/chronic-sleep-disturbance-might-trigger-onset-alzheimer%E2%80%99s>.

Morgan, P.J., et al. "The impact of a workplace-based weight loss program on work-related outcomes in overweight male shift workers." *Journal of Occupational and Environmental Medicine / American College of Occupational and Environmental Medicine* 54.2 (2012): 122-127. PubMed.gov. 20 Jan. 2015. <http://www.ncbi.nlm.nih.gov/pubmed/22269987>.

Mullaney, Rebekah. "Depending on How Much and How Long, Light from Self-Luminous Tablet Computers Can Affect Evening Melatonin, Delaying Sleep." *Lighting Research Center: Press Releases* 21 Aug. 2012. 18 Jan. 2015. <http://www.lrc.rpi.edu/resources/newsroom/pr_story.asp?id=235#.VLycCZUtHIU>.

Mutungi, Gisella, et al. "Dietary Cholesterol from Eggs Increases Plasma HDL Cholesterol in Overweight Men Consuming a Carbohydrate-Restricted Diet." *Journal of Nutrition* 138.2 (2008): 272-276. 14 Jan. 2015. <http://jn.nutrition.org/content/138/2/272.abstract>.

Myllymäki T., et al. "Effects of vigorous late-night exercise on sleep quality and cardiac autonomic activity." *Journal of Sleep Research* 20.1 Pt 2 (2011): 146-153. PubMed.gov. 18 Jan. 2015. <http://www.ncbi.nlm.nih.gov/pubmed/20673290>.

"Napping may not be such a no-no." *Harvard Health Publications: Harvard Medical School* Nov. 2009. 17 Jan. 2015. <http://www.health.harvard.edu/newsletters/Harvard_Health_Letter/2009/November/napping-may-not-be-such-a-no-no>.

"National Walking Day: 5 Ways Walking Helps To Relieve Stress." *HuffPost: Healthy Living* 3 April 2013. 22 Jan. 2015. <http://www.huffingtonpost.com/2013/04/03/national-walking-day-stress-relief-tips_n_2992972.html>.

Neal, David T., Wendy Wood, and Aimme Drolet. "How do people adhere to goals when willpower is low? The profits (and pitfalls) of strong habits." *Journal of Personality and Social Psychology* 104.6 (2013): 959-975. APA PsychNET. 24 Jan. 2015. <http://psycnet.apa.org/journals/psp/104/6/959/>.

Nelson, Jennifer. "Clear the Clutter Out of Your Life." *WebMD* 29 June 2010. 22 Jan. 2015. <http://www.webmd.com/balance/features/clear-clutter-out-your-life?page=3>.

Neporent, Liz. "Crash Test Dummies Gain Weight to Save Lives." *ABC News* 29 Oct. 2014. 17 Jan. 2015. <http://abcnews.go.com/Health/fat-ter-crash-test-dummies-prevent-road-deaths/story?id=26545335>.

"New Survey: To Sit or Stand? Almost 70% of Full Time American Workers Hate Sitting, but They do it all Day Every Day." *PR Newswire* 17 July 2013. 18 Jan. 2015. <http://www.prnewswire.com/news-releases/new-survey-to-sit-or-stand-almost-70-of-full-time-american-workers-hate-sitting-but-they-do-it-all-day-every-day-215804771.html>.

"News & Research: Facts at a Glance." *National Restaurant Association* 16 Jan. 2015. 17 Jan. 2015. <http://www.restaurant.org/News-Research/Research/Facts-at-a-Glance>.

"News: Coffee by the Numbers." *Harvard T.H. Chan School of Public Health* 14 Jan. 2015. <http://www.hsph.harvard.edu/news/multimedia-article/facts/>.

"NHTSA, Virginia Tech Transportation Institute Release Findings of Breakthrough Research on Real-World Driver Behavior, Distraction and Crash Factors." *National Highway Traffic Safety Administration* 20 Apr. 2006. 17 Jan. 2015. <http://www.nhtsa.gov/Driving+Safety/Distracted+Driving+at+Distraction.gov/Breakthrough+Research+on+-Real-World+Driver+Behavior+Released>.

Norton, Amy. "Working Night Shift May Slow Your Metabolism." *WebMD* 18 Nov. 2014. 17 Jan. 2015. <http://www.webmd.com/diet/news/20141118/working-night-shift-slows-metabolism-study-suggests>.

O'Connor, Anahad. "The Claim: Spicy Foods Increase Metabolism." *The New York Times* 28 Nov. 2006. 18 Jan. 2015. <http://www.nytimes.com/2006/11/28/health/nutrition/28real.html?_r=1&>.

Park, Alice. "12 Breakfast Cereals That Are More Than 50% Sugar." *Time* 15 May 2014. 13 Jan. 2015. <http://time.com/97714/cereals-contain-50-sugar-by-weight/>.

Parker-Pope, Tara. "Well: The Risks and Rewards of Skipping Meals." *The New York Times* 26 Dec. 2007. 15 Jan. 2015. <http://well.blogs.nytimes.com/2007/12/26/the-risks-and-rewards-of-skipping-meals/?_r=0>.

Parker-Pope, Tara. "Workplace Cited as a New Source of Rise in Obesity." *The New York Times* 26 May 2011. 20 Jan. 2015. <http://www.nytimes.com/2011/05/26/health/nutrition/26fat.html?pagewanted=all >.

"Partners in Weight Loss Success May Help African-Americans Shed More Pounds." *Penn Medicine: News & Publications* 7 Oct. 2009. 18 Jan. 2015. <http://www.uphs.upenn.edu/news/News_Releases/2009/10/partners-in-weight-loss/>.

Patel, S.R., et al. "Association between reduced sleep and weight gain in women." *American Journal of Epidemiology* 164.10 (2006): 947-954. PubMed.gov. 18 Jan. 2015. <http://www.ncbi.nlm.nih.gov/pubmed/16914506?dopt=Citation>.

Pathe, Simone. "The secret to improving health and productivity at work." *PBS NEWSHOUR* 12 March 2014. 20 Jan. 2015. <http://www.pbs.org/newshour/making-sense/secret-improving-health-productivity-work/>.

Payne, Emily. "Is your caffeine fix making you fat? Study shows five cups of coffee a day could cause obesity." *Daily Mail* 28 May 2013. 17 Jan. 2015. <http://www.dailymail.co.uk/health/article-2332044/Is-caffeine-fix-making-fat-Study-shows-cups-coffee-day-cause-obesity.html>.

"Penn Medicine Researchers Show How Lost Sleep Leads to Lost Neurons." *Penn Medicine: News & Publications* 18 Mar. 2014. 19 Jan. 2015. <http://www.uphs.upenn.edu/news/news_releases/2014/03/veasey/>.

Peri, Camille. "Coping With Excessive Sleepiness: How to Stay Awake Naturally." *WebMD* 17 Feb. 2012. 17 Jan. 2015. <http://www.webmd.com/sleep-disorders/excessive-sleepiness-10/natural-tips-sleepiness>.

Perry-Jenkins, Maureen, et al. "Shift Work, Role Overload, and the Transition to Parenthood." *Journal of Marriage and the Family* 69.1 (2007):

123-138. PMC. 24 Jan. 2015. <http://www.ncbi.nlm.nih.gov/pmc/articles/PMC2834316/>.

"Phytosterols: Sterols & Stanols." *Cleveland Clinic* Oct. 2013. 14 Jan. 2015. <http://my.clevelandclinic.org/services/heart/prevention/nutrition/food-choices/phytosterols-sterols-stanols>.

Picco, Michael F. "Nutrition and healthy eating: Does drinking water during or after a meal disturb digestion?" *Mayo Clinic* 19 Apr. 2012. 19 Jan. 2015. <http://www.mayoclinic.org/healthy-living/nutrition-and-healthy-eating/expert-answers/digestion/faq-20058348>.

Polis, Carey. "31 Million Americans Skip Breakfast Each Day." *Huff-Post: Food* 11 Oct. 2011. 5 Jan. 2015. <http://www.huffingtonpost.com/2011/10/11/31-million-americans-skip_n_1005076.html>.

Pollack, Andrew. "Business Day: A.M.A. Recognizes Obesity as a Disease." *The New York Times* 18 June 2013. 12 Jan 2015. <http://www.nytimes.com/2013/06/19/business/ama-recognizes-obesity-as-a-disease.html>.

"Q&A on Stress for Adults: How it affects your health and what you can do about it." *National Institute of Mental Health* 22 Jan. 2015. <http://www.nimh.nih.gov/health/publications/stress/index.shtml>.

Rampersaud, G.C., et al. "Breakfast habits, nutritional status, body weight, and academic performance in children and adolescents." *Journal of the American Dietetic Association* 105.5 (2005): 743-762. PubMed.gov. 13 Jan. 2015. <http://www.ncbi.nlm.nih.gov/pubmed/15883552>.

Ratini, Melinda. "Are You Getting Enough Sleep?" *WebMD* 16 May 2014. 18 Jan. 2015. <http://www.webmd.com/sleep-disorders/guide/sleep-requirements>.

Reaney, Patricia. "Long commutes may be bad for health: study." *Reuters* 8 May 2012. 17 Jan. 2015. <http://www.reuters.com/article/2012/05/08/us-commuting-idUSBRE8470U520120508>.

Rebello, C.J., et al. "Acute effect of oatmeal on subjective measures of appetite and satiety compared to a ready-to-eat breakfast cereal: a randomized crossover trial." *Journal of the American College of Nutrition* 34.2 (2013): 272-279. PubMed.gov. 14 Jan. 2015. <http://www.ncbi.nlm.nih.gov/pubmed/24024772>.

Rettner, Rachael. "Obese Employees Take More Sick Leave." *Live Science* 2 Aug. 2010. 12 Jan. 2015. <http://www.livescience.com/6819-obese-employees-sick-leave.html>.

Rettner, Rachael. "The Truth About '10,000 Steps' a Day." *Live Science* 7 Mar. 2014. 23 Jan. 2015. <http://www.livescience.com/43956-walking-10000-steps-healthy.html>.

Reuteman, Rob. "Vocational School Enrollment Booms Amid White-Collar Bust." *CNBC* 3 Dec. 2009. 24 Jan. 2015. <http://www.cnbc.com/id/34256312#.>.

Reuters. "Airline says pay-by-weight is 'fairest' way to fly." *Chicago Tribune* 3 Apr. 2013. 16 Jan. 2015. <http://articles.chicagotribune.com/2013-04-03/business/chi-airlines-says-paybyweight-plan-is-fairest-way-to-fly-20130403_1_fairest-way-american-samoa-obese-passengers>.

Robehmed, Natalie. "Healthy Vending Machines: The Future of Snack Foods." *Forbes* 27 July 2012. 17 Jan. 2015. <http://www.forbes.com/sites/natalierobehmed/2012/07/27/healthy-vending-machines-the-future-of-snack-food/>.

Rones, Nancy. "Health & Balance: Your Guide To Never Feeling Tired Again." *WebMD* 1 Mar. 2007. 17 Jan. 2015. <http://www.webmd.com/balance/features/your-guide-to-never-feeling-tired-again>.

Rouhani, M. H., et al. "Is there a relationship between red or processed meat intake and obesity? A systematic review and meta-analysis of observational studies." *Obesity Reviews* 15.9 (2014) 740-748. Wiley Online Library. 13 Jan. 2015. <http://onlinelibrary.wiley.com/doi/10.1111/obr.12172/abstract>.

Saad, Lydia. "The "40-Hour" Work Week Is Actually Longer—by Seven Hours." *Gallup* 29 Aug. 2014. 18 Jan. 2015. <http://www.gallup.com/poll/175286/hour-workweek-actually-longer-seven-hours.aspx>.

Sarnataro, Barbara Russi. "Fitness Basics: Swimming Is For Everyone." *WebMD* 16 Jan. 2015. <http://www.webmd.com/fitness-exercise/features/fitness-basics-swimming-is-for-everyone>.

Sauter, Steven, et al. "STRESS...At Work." *Centers for Disease Control and Prevention* DHHS (NIOSH) 99-101 (1999). 21 Jan. 2015. <http://www.cdc.gov/niosh/docs/99-101/>.

Schmidt, Elaine. "This is your brain on sugar: UCLA study shows high fructose diet sabotages learning, memory." *UCLA Newsroom* 15 May 2012. 13 Jan. 2015. <http://newsroom.ucla.edu/releases/this-is-your-brain-on-sugar-ucla-233992>.

Schulte, Brigid. "U.S. productivity: Putting in all those hours doesn't matter." *The Washington Post* 14 May 2014. 18 Jan. 2015. <http://www.washingtonpost.com/blogs/she-the-people/wp/2014/05/14/u-s-productivity-putting-in-all-those-hours-doesnt-matter/>.

Schwartz, Tony. "Relax! You'll Be More Productive." *The New York Times* 9 Feb. 2013. 18 Jan. 2015. <http://www.nytimes.com/2013/02/10/opinion/sunday/relax-youll-be-more-productive.html?pagewanted=all&_r=2&>.

Seliger, Susan. "'Superfoods' Everyone Needs." *WebMD* 16 February 2007. 20 Jan. 2015. <http://www.webmd.com/diet/features/superfoods-everyone-needs>.

Shah, Yagana. "Just 15 Minutes of Exercise A Day Can Lower Your Risk of Breast Cancer, Study Says." *HuffPost: Huff50* 3 Nov. 2014. 16 Jan. 2015. <http://www.huffingtonpost.com/2014/11/03/exercise-lowers-breast-cancer-risk_n_6094658.html>.

Shaw, Gina. "Water and Stress Reduction: Sipping Stress Away." *WebMD* 7 July 2009. 17 Jan. 2015. <http://www.webmd.com/diet/features/water-stress-reduction>.

Schocker, Laura. "This Is Your Body On Stress (INFOGRAPHIC)." *Huffpost: Healthy Living* 5 April 2013. 21 Jan. 2015. <http://www.huffingtonpost.com/2013/03/19/body-stress-response_n_2902073.html>.

"Shocking Benefits of Exercising on an Empty Stomach." *HuffPost: Healthy Living* 24 June 2014. 15 Jan. 2015. <http://www.huffingtonpost.com/the-active-times/shocking-benefits-of-exer_b_5207788.html>.

"Sitting At Work: Why It's Dangerous And What You Can Do." *HuffPost: Healthy Living* 30 June 2014. 19 Jan. 2015. <http://www.huffingtonpost.com/2012/07/24/sitting-at-work-why-its-dangerous-alternatives_n_1695618.html>.

"Sleep More, Weigh Less." *WebMD* 30 June 2014. 17 Jan. 2015. <http://www.webmd.com/diet/sleep-and-weight-loss>.

Smith, A.P. "Breakfast and mental health." *International Journal of Food Sciences and Nutrition* 5 (1998): 397-402. PubMed.gov. 13 Jan. 2015. <http://www.ncbi.nlm.nih.gov/pubmed/10367010>.

Smith, Jacquelyn. "The 10 Best Exercises To Do At Your Desk." *Forbes* 6 Feb. 2013. 20 Jan. 2015. <http://www.forbes.com/sites/jacquelynsmith/2013/02/06/the-10-best-exercises-to-do-at-your-desk/>.

"Snacking While Driving: Top 10 Foods To Stay Away From." *Huff-Post: Teen* 18 Dec. 2011. 17 Jan. 2015. <http://www.huffingtonpost.com/2011/10/18/snacking-while-driving-to_n_1017394.html>.

Söderström M., et al. "Insufficient Sleep Predicts Clinical Burnout." *Journal of Occupational Health Psychology* 17.2 (2012): 175-183. PubMed.gov. 18 Jan. 2015. <http://www.ncbi.nlm.nih.gov/pubmed/22449013>.

Soong, Jennifer. "The Secret (and Surprising) Power of Naps." *WebMD* 29 Nov. 2011. 22 Jan. 2015. <http://www.webmd.com/balance/features/the-secret-and-surprising-power-of-naps>.

Squires, Sally. "Drive Yourself To Fitness." *The Washington Post* 15 Aug. 2006. 17 Jan. 2015. <http://www.washingtonpost.com/wp-dyn/content/article/2006/08/14/AR2006081400879.html>.

"Stand Up, Walk Around, Even Just For '20 Minutes.'" *NPR.org* 9 May 2012. 19 Jan. 2015. <http://www.npr.org/2012/05/09/152336802/stand-up-walk-around-even-just-for-20-minutes>.

Stewart, Hayden, et al. "Economic Research Service: The Demand for Food Away From Home: Full Service or Fast Food?" *United States Department of Agriculture* Jan. 2004. Agricultural Economic Report No. 829. 18 Jan. 2015. <http://www.ers.usda.gov/media/306585/aer829_1_.pdf>.

Stott-Miller, Marni, Marian L. Neuhouser, and Janet L. Stanford. "Consumption of deep-fried foods and risk of prostate cancer." *The Prostate* 73.9 (2013): 960-969. Wiley Online Library. 12 Jan. 2015. <http://onlinelibrary.wiley.com/doi/10.1002/pros.22643/abstract>.

"Stress Interferes with Problem-Solving; Beta-Blocker May Help." *Ohio State Research News* 9 Nov. 2005. 21 Jan. 2015. <http://researchnews.osu.edu/archive/strsbeta.htm>.

"Stress Management: Breathing Exercises for Relaxation." *WebMD* 15 May 2012. 22 Jan. 2015. <http://www.webmd.com/balance/stress-management/stress-management-breathing-exercises-for-relaxation>.

"Stress Management: Doing Progressive Muscle Relaxation." *WebMD* 15 May 2012. 23 Jan. 2015. <http://www.webmd.com/balance/stress-<management/stress-management-doing-progressive-muscle-relaxation>.

Stromberg, Joseph. "Five Health Benefits of Standing Desks." *Smithsonian.com* 26 March 2014. 20 Jan 2015. <http://www.smithsonianmag.com/science-nature/five-health-benefits-standing-desks-180950259/?no-ist>.

Stump, Scott. "'Nap rooms' encourage sleeping on the job to boost productivity." *Today: Money* 15 Mar. 2013. 17 Jan. 2015. <http://www.today.com/money/nap-rooms-encourage-sleeping-job-boost-productivity-1C8881304>.

Sugiyama T., D. Ding, and N. Owen. "Commuting by car: weight gain among physically active adults." *American Journal of Preventive Medicine* 44.2 (2013): 169-173. PubMed.gov. 17 Jan. 2015. <http://www.ncbi.nlm.nih.gov/pubmed/23332335>.

Swartz, Ann M., et al. "Prompts to Disrupt Sitting Time and Increase Physical Activity at Work, 2011-2012." *Preventing Chronic Disease* 130318.11 (2014). Centers for Disease Control and Prevention. 20 Jan. 2015. <http://www.cdc.gov/pcd/issues/2014/13_0318.htm>.

Tanchoco, Celeste C., et al. "The Effect of Egg Consumption on Lipid Profile Among Selected 30-60 Year-Old Filipino Adults." *Philippine Journal of Science* 140.1 (2011): 51-58. 14 Jan. 2015. <http://philjournalsci.dost.gov.ph/vol140no1/pdfs/7_the%20effect%20of%20egg%20consumption%20on%20lipid%20profile%20among%20selected%20filipino%20adults.pdf>.

Tarkan, Laurie. "Another Reason Not To Skip Lunch." *CBS News* 18 Aug. 2011. 15 Jan. 2015. <http://www.cbsnews.com/news/another-reason-not-to-skip-lunch/>.

"Tea and Cancer Prevention: Strengths and Limits of the Evidence." *National Cancer Institute* Nov. 17 2010. 14 Jan. 2015. <http://www.cancer.gov/cancertopics/factsheet/prevention/tea>.

"The Benefits of Walking." *American Heart Association* 15 Jan. 2015. <http://www.startwalkingnow.org/whystart_benefits_walking.jsp>.

"The Health Benefits of Yoga." *WebMD* 24 June 2014. 23 Jan. 2015. <http://www.webmd.com/balance/guide/the-health-benefits-of-yoga>.

"The Micro-skills of Non-verbal Language." *AIPC Article Library* 22 Mar. 2012. 20 Jan. 2015. <http://www.aipc.net.au/articles/the-micro-skills-of-non-verbal-language/>.

"The New (Ab)Normal: Portion Sizes Today vs. In The 1950s (INFOGRAPHIC)." *HuffPost: Healthy Living* 23 May 2012. 15 Jan. 2015. <http://www.huffingtonpost.com/2012/05/23/portion-sizes-infographic_n_1539804.html>.

"The Nutrition Source: Healthy Gains from Whole Grains." *Harvard T.H. Chan School of Public Health* 14 Jan. 2015. <http://www.hsph.harvard.edu/nutritionsource/what-should-you-eat/health-gains-from-whole-grains/>.

"The Nutrition Source: Sleep Deprivation and Obesity." *Harvard T.H. Chan School of Public Health* 18 Jan. 2015. <http://www.hsph.harvard.edu/nutritionsource/sleep/#2>.

"The Nutrition Source: Top Food Sources of Saturated Fat In The U.S." *Harvard T.H. Chan School of Public Health* 18 Jan. 2015. <http://www.hsph.harvard.edu/nutritionsource/top-food-sources-of-saturated-fat-in-the-us/>.

"Transportation Security Administration: Food and Beverages." *Department of Homeland Security* 27 Jan. 2014. 16 Jan. 2015. <http://www.tsa.gov/traveler-information/food-and-beverages>.

Trappe, Hans-Joachim. "The effects of music on the cardiovascular system and cardiovascular health." *Heart* 96 (2010): 1868-1871. 17 Jan. 2015. <http://heart.bmj.com/content/96/23/1868>.

Turner, Ashley. "Lonely or Hungry... How to Deal with Emotional Eating." *HuffPost: Healthy Living* 5 Aug. 2013. 16 Jan. 2015. <http://www.huffingtonpost.com/ashley-turner/emotional-eating_b_3705430.html>.

University of California - San Diego. "Let Me Sleep On It: Creative Problem Solving Enhanced By REM Sleep." *ScienceDaily* 9 June 2009. 17 Jan. 2015. <www.sciencedaily.com/releases/2009/06/090608182421.htm>.

University of Georgia. "Low-intensity Exercise Reduces Fatigue Symptoms By 65 Percent, Study Finds." *ScienceDaily* 2 March 2008. 24 Jan. 2015. <www.sciencedaily.com/releases/2008/02/080228112008.htm>.

"Unraveling the Sun's Role in Depression." *WebMD* 5 Dec. 2002. 17 Jan. 2015. <http://www.webmd.com/mental-health/news/20021205/unraveling-suns-role-in-depression>.

Vander Wal, J.S., et al. "Egg breakfast enhances weight loss" *International Journal of Obesity (Lond)* 32.10 (2008): 1545-1551. PMC. 14 Jan. 2015. <http://www.ncbi.nlm.nih.gov/pmc/articles/PMC2755181/>.

Vander Wal, J.S., et al. "Short-term effect of eggs on satiety in overweight and obese subjects." *Journal of the American College of Nutrition* 24.6 (2005): 510-515. PubMed.gov. 13 Jan. 2015. <http://www.ncbi.nlm.nih.gov/pubmed/16373948>.

Vlahos, James. "Is Sitting a Lethal Activity?" *The New York Times* 14 Apr. 2011. 18 Jan. 2015. <http://www.nytimes.com/2011/04/17/magazine/mag-17sitting-t.html?_r=0>.

Wallheimer, Brian. "Purdue University News Service: Red wine, fruit compound could help block fat cell formation." *Purdue University* 4 Apr. 2012. 18 Jan. 2015. <http://www.purdue.edu/newsroom/research/2012/120404KimPiceatannol.html>.

Wansink, B. "Environmental factors that increase the food intake and consumption volume of unknowing consumers." *Annual Review of Nutrition* 24 (2004): 455-479. PubMed.gov. 25 Jan. 2015. <http://www.ncbi.nlm.nih.gov/pubmed/15189128.>.

Wansink, Brian, and Koert van Ittersum. "The Visual Illusions of Food: Why Plates, Bowls, and Spoons Can Bias Consumption Volume." *The Journal of the Federation of American Societies for Experimental Biology* 20.A618. (2006). 18 Jan. 2015. <http://www.fasebj.org/cgi/content/meeting_abstract/20/4/A618-c>.

Warner, Jennifer. "Stress Feeds the Need for Comfort Food." *WebMD* 9 Sept. 2003. 21 Jan. 2015. <http://www.webmd.com/balance/news/20030909/stress-comfort-food>.

Warner, Jennifer. "Substance Abuse and Addiction Health Center: Loud Bar Music Makes You Drink More." *WebMD* 18 July 2008. 18 Jan. 2015. <http://www.webmd.com/mental-health/addiction/news/20080718/loud-bar-music-makes-you-drink-more>.

Waterlow, Lucy. "Revealed: The tricks fast food restaurants use to get you to eat more." *Daily Mail* 13 Jan. 2014. 17 Jan. 2015. <http://www.dailymail.co.uk/femail/article-2538568/REVEALED-The-tricks-fast-food-restaurants-use-eat-more.html>.

"Weight loss and breakfast : Breakfast benefits health and can aid in weight loss." *Harvard Health Publications: Harvard Medical School* Feb. 2005. 14 Jan. 2015. <http://www.health.harvard.edu/press_releases/weight_loss_healthy_breakfast>.

Weiss, Tara. "The advantages to working the graveyard shift." *Forbes.com on NBCNews.com* 7 April 2008. 17 Jan. 2015. <http://www.nbcnews.com/id/23676757/ns/business-forbes_com/t/advantages-working-graveyard-shift/#.VLreVpUtHIU>.

"What is it about coffee?" *Harvard Health Publications: Harvard Medical School* 1 Jan. 2012. <http://www.health.harvard.edu/press_releases/what-is-it-about-coffee>.

"What is the relationship between whole grain intake and body weight?" *United States Department of Agriculture* Nutrition Evidence Library.gov. 14 Jan. 2015. <http://www.nel.gov/evidence.cfm?evidence_summary_id=250304>.

"Why lack of sleep is bad for your health." *NHS: Choices* 18 June 2013. 18 Jan. 2015. <http://www.nhs.uk/livewell/tiredness-and-fatigue/pages/lack-of-sleep-health-risks.aspx>.

Wong, May. "Stanford study finds walking improves creativity." *Stanford Report* 24 Apr. 2014. 19 Jan. 2015. <http://news.stanford.edu/news/2014/april/walking-vs-sitting-042414.html>.

"Work Stress On The Rise: 8 In 10 Americans Are Stressed About Their Jobs, Survey Finds." *HuffPost: Healthy Living* 12 Apr. 2013. 21 Jan. 2015 <http://www.huffingtonpost.com/2013/04/10/work-stress-jobs-americans_n_3053428.html>.

"Workplace Health Promotion: Increase Productivity." *Centers for Disease Control and Prevention* 23 Oct. 2013. 12 Jan. 2015. <http://www.cdc.gov/workplacehealthpromotion/businesscase/benefits/productivity.html>.

"Workplace Stress." *The American Institute of Stress* 21 Jan. 2015. <http://www.stress.org/workplace-stress/>.

Zamosky, Lisa. "The Truth about Tryptophan." *WebMD* 18 Nov. 2009. 17 Jan. 2015. <http://www.webmd.com/food-recipes/features/the-truth-about-tryptophan?page=3>.

Zelman, Kathleen M. "6 Reasons to Drink Water." *WebMD* 8 May 2008. 15 Jan. 2015. <http://www.webmd.com/diet/features/6-reasons-to-drink-water>.

Zelman, Kathleen M. "Diet Truth or Myth: Eating at Night Causes Weight Gain." *WebMD* 8 Sept. 2011. 18 Jan. 2015. <http://www.webmd.com/diet/features/diet-truth-myth-eating-night-causes-weight-gain>.

Zelman, Kathleen M. "Low-Calorie Cocktails." *WebMD* 18 July 2011. 18 Jan. 2015. <http://www.webmd.com/diet/features/low-calorie-cocktails>.

Zelman, Kathleen M. "The Many Benefits of Breakfast." *WebMD* 29 Aug. 2007. 13 Jan. 2015. <http://www.webmd.com/diet/features/many-benefits-breakfast>.

Zelman, Kathleen M. "What to Eat Before, During, and After Exercise." *WebMD* 19 June 2013. 18 Jan. 2015. <http://www.webmd.com/diet/features/what-eat-before-during-after-exercise>.

Zuckerbrot, Tanya. "The Truth About Bagels." *Fox News Magazine* 21 Sept. 2012. 12 Jan. 2015. <http://magazine.foxnews.com/food-wellness/truth-about-bagels>.

Index

chicken
  breakfast ideas, 31
  and telecommuting, 189
  and conferences, 175
  and eating out, 109, 170, 219
  from coworkers, 17
  if you cook, 216
  if you don't cook, 217
  lunch, 102–105
  at lunch-and-learns, 130
  on pizza, 228
  and shift workers, 199–200,
      227–228
  post workout, 44
  and potluck, 107
  and food industry employees,
      204, 206
children
  and breakfast, 29–30
  in the kitchen, 18
  and pre-work commitments, 60
  and night shift employees, 193
  at workplace, 6
  and your weight goals, 198
Children's Hospital of
    Pennsylvania, 139
chips
  chocolate, 18, 121
  kale, 216
  pita, 198
  potato, 106, 129, 167–168,
      186, 192, 212, 214, 227
  tortilla, 103
cholesterol
  and breakfast, 26, 28, 30, 33

  and chronic stress, 143
  and commuting, 46
  count, 5
  and eggs, 31
  and exercise, 43
  HDL, 11, 31, 37
  and health fair screenings, 136
  LDL, 11, 33–34, 72, 223
  and prolonged sitting, 72
  and tea, 37
  and whole grains, 34
  and red wine, 223
cinnamon, 12, 14, 27, 61, 163–164
clutter, cutting, 158–159
coconut water, 41
coffee, 1–2, 12, 35–37, 39, 41–42,
    100, 172–173, 192, 201, 229
coffee cake, 12, 14, 207
comfort foods, 50, 52, 143, 145, 152
commitment to weight loss, xvii,
    21, 113–114, 124, 179, 231
commuting
  biking options, 63–65
  and boredom, 66
  destressing, 58–61
  and eating, 61–63
  and exercising, 51–58, 65
  fast food, 50–51
  managing the ride, 66–67
  precautions, 67–68
  prolonged sitting, 48–49
  statistics, 45
  stressors, 49–50
  time reduced for other
      activities, 49

and commuting, 47, 49,
    51–59, 65
and contracts with yourself, 29
and eating, 43–44
and food industry employees,
    205
and health fairs, 136–137
and lunch, 109
and stress, 156–157
tailored to your schedule, 43
and telecommuting, 189–190
in today's workplaces, xvi
and traveling, 175–177
and walking, 135
and weight gain, 49, 70–71
after work, 229–234
and yoga, 137–138
at your desk, 80–92

F
fast food
    breakfast, 39–40
    and commuting, 50–51, 62–63
    cost of, 41–42
    and food industry employees,
        202
    frequency of consuming,
        209–210, 218
    at home, 219–220
    and lunch, 95, 98, 108
    and night shift employees, 192
    and recognition, 119
    and traveling, 164–165
fat, body
    and your job, xv, xvii, xix

burning fat, 43
and commuting, 47–48, 51,
    54, 62–63
and desk dining, 98
food trucks, 110–111
and furniture, 87
and happy hours, 224
and long hours, 226–227
and sleeping, 235–236
and sitting, 71
and stress, 147
and traveling, 175
fat-free, 13–14, 107, 129
fats. *See also* fat-free; low-fat
    options; nonfat options
    bagels, 10
    and breakfast, 23, 27–28,
        39–40
    and cinnamon buns, 12
    and coffee, 36
    coworkers treats, 15–21
    cutting them down, 13
    donuts, 10–11
    and events, 117, 120–124, 242
    facts, 28
    and fast food, 164–166
    and food industry employees,
        206
    and frozen yogurt, 107, 166
    and lunch, 102–103, 108
    at lunch-and-learns, 129–130
    and night shift employees, 200
    and pizza, 228
    and potlucks, 106
    and recognition, 132

replacing, 34
and restaurant food, 217–220
and red wine, 223
and sleeping, 235–236
and sweet rolls, 12
and technology, 211
and your weight loss goals, 6
across the workplace, 1, 3, 5–6
fatty acids, 103
feedback, 80, 119–120, 134, 184–185, 205
fiber, 10, 30–35, 38, 102, 114, 166, 199–201
finger food, 5–6
flour, 11, 18, 34
food service employees, 182, 202–208
food trucks, 110–111
fried foods, 10, 15, 17, 163, 175, 204, 219, 222
frozen foods, 40–41, 105, 107, 166, 200, 217, 227
fruit
    at breakfast, 32, 38–39
    and commuting, 62
    at conferences, 175
    at conventions, 172–173
    on cruises, 180
    as company food offerings, 15
    at company-sponsored events, 129–130
    as dessert, 220
    dried, 5, 32, 127
    and food industry jobs, 204, 206

juices, 34–35, 105, 172–173
at lunch, 102, 105, 109
and morning workouts, 44
and the night shift, 199, 201
and per diem meals, 170
and potlucks, 107
recipes, 41
serving size, 214
and snacking, 114
and traveling, 166, 168

G
Gallup Poll, 209, 234
gastroesophageal reflux disease (GERD), 36
gifts, of food, 15, 18, 21–22, 207
glucose, 99, 142, 146–147
gluten-free, 14, 175, 198
goals, exercise, 43, 57, 72, 135, 230
goals, walking, 134–135
goals, weight loss
    and alcohol, 168, 177, 223
    and breakfast, 31, 38–39
    and the candy bowl, 6
    commitment to achieve, xvii
    and commuting, 62
    and dinner, 200, 216
    and your family and friends, 198
    and company events, 120, 124, 131
    and cruises, 179–180
    eating out, 220–221
    establishing, 4–5, 241
    and food industry employees, 203–204, 206

and food trucks, 111
and the night shift, 190, 194
and ordering food, 227–228
and pizza, 227–228
positive messages, 92
post-work eating, 214–215
potlucks, at work, 106–107
pursuing, 13
and saboteurs, 20
and sleeping, 238
and stress management,
    147–148
and telecommuting, 185,
    187, 189
and trans fats, 11, 13, 129
and traveling, 163, 170
goals, work, 9, 13, 76, 133,
    164–165, 178–179, 241
guided imagery, 161

H
happy hours, 210, 222–224
Harris Interactive, 140
Harvard Division of Sleep
    Medicine, 194–195
Harvard Health Letter, 36
Harvard University, 26, 28, 31,
    97, 237
health fair, 136–137
healthy bars, 5, 38, 62, 166,
    198, 230
heart disease
    and breakfast blunders,
        27–28
    and cereal choices, 31–32

and commuting, 46
and fast food, 164
and Mediterranean diet, 130
and night shift work, 191
and prolonged sitting, 49, 72
and skipping breakfast, 26
and sleep deprivation, 236
and stress, 143
and tea, 37
and trans fats, 11, 13, 129
and walking, 112
and whole wheat and whole
    grain selections, 34
holidays, 118–119, 123, 128
hummus, 13, 103, 106, 224
hunger
    fruit, 204
    and hydration, 62, 203–204
    managing, 21, 100, 115, 212,
        214–215
    and night shift, 199
    pay attention to, 7
    protein and fiber, 30
    and skipping breakfast, 26
    snacks, 199, 230
    after work, 230–231
hypertension, 37, 43, 72
hypothalamus, 142

I
ice cream, 119–123, 140, 147,
    186, 212
insulin, 26, 36, 99
International Journal of Obesity,
    226

and planning and time, 37–39,
42, 62, 101–102, 113,
131, 238
and sleeping, 238–239
and stress, 58–59, 142–143
147–149, 152–162
and weight, 6, 21, 30, 33,
40, 73, 76–77, 91, 115,
164–165, 181, 199, 205,
213, 230, 242
wandering around, 79–80
Manager. *See* management
Managing. *See* management
Mayo Clinic, 70, 90, 156, 168
McMaster University, 86
measurement, xvii, 4, 10, 13, 32,
68, 72, 89, 91, 133–134, 148,
152, 161, 165, 201, 214, 216,
220, 242
meditation, 156–157, 240
Mediterranean diet, 130
meetings, xvi–xvii, 7, 69, 75–76,
87, 95, 112, 115, 121, 163,
183–184, 211, 230, 237, 239
melatonin, 235
menus
breakfast, 39
and out-of-home dining,
219–221, 227
and events, 119, 124–125, 128
lunch, 108–110
traveling, 165–166, 170–171,
174
metabolism, 71, 84, 99–100, 228
Metabolism, 99–100

milk, 32, 35, 39, 147, 169, 172, 239
motivation, 16, 20, 92, 115,
118–120, 127, 132–133, 141,
187–188, 226, 229–231, 232
muffins, 23, 33, 40, 55, 62, 172, 207
muscle relaxation, 160
music
and commuting, 50, 59
and exercise, 190
and energy, 197, 229
and happy hours, 222
and stress management, 162
and traveling, 169

N
NASA, 159
napping, 159, 194–195, 196–197,
229
National Highway Traffic Safety
Administration, 67
National Sleep Foundation, 234
*New England Journal of
Medicine*, 36
Nielsen survey, 49
night shift work, 190–201
nonfat options, 13, 32, 38, 39–40,
129
Northwestern University, 191
nuts, 5, 15, 32, 34, 40–41, 44, 62,
105, 114, 127, 130, 166, 169,
189, 200–201, 222, 224, 230, 239

O
oatmeal, 25, 33, 39, 172–173, 189

obesity
and caffeine, 229
and commuting, 47, 49, 52
epidemic, xvi, xviii, xix
and exercise, 43
and food choices, 27–28, 30, 34, 218
and illness, xix
and night shift, 191
skipping meals, 23, 25, 99
and sleeping, 236
and traveling, 164, 179
and walking, 112
objectives. *See* goals
Office for National Statistics and the Center for Economics and Business Research, 27
OfficeTeam, 94
Ohio State University Medical Center, 144
omega-3, 33, 103
opportunity binge, 164
overeating, 97–100, 102–104, 106–107, 112, 179, 203, 212, 214, 220, 224
overtime, 209, 225–227
overweight, xvi, xviii, 30–31, 90, 218, 225

P
parking, 7, 63–64, 79, 80, 109, 136
parties, xviii, 177–178, 242
peanut butter, 34, 230
pedometers, 90, 133–136

peer pressure, 3, 19–21, 96, 106–108, 126, 182, 203
Pennington Biomedical Research Center, 30–31
Pennsylvania State University, 228–229
peppermint, 61
per diem allowance, 170–172
phone, xvi–xvii, 6, 24, 29, 59, 67, 69, 73–74, 77, 95, 111–112, 165, 174, 183, 194, 211–212, 235
physical activity. *See* exercise
phytosterols, 34
Pilates, 43, 177, 231–232
pizza, xviii, 129, 192, 201, 228–229
planning. *See also* management; strategies
and commuting, 48, 60, 62–63, 68
and events, 122, 124–126, 137
implementation, 4, 29, 33, 37–38, 39, 42, 215, 221–222, 224, 227, 230, 241–242
and stress management, 147–148, 154
and travel, 163–170, 173, 178, 180
and unconventional jobs, 189, 194, 199–200, 205
and weight control, xvii, 7, 22, 39, 48, 73, 77, 100–101, 103–104, 112, 115
PLoS One, xvi

portions, 1, 14, 32–33, 97,
101, 104, 107, 112, 114,
125, 212–214, 216, 218,
220–221, 224
potassium, 33, 38
potlucks, 105–108
pounds
and alcohol consumption,
167–168, 221–222
and breakfast, 28, 39
and commuting, 45, 67–68
and dinner, 209, 215
exercise, 231
and feedback, 120, 132
goals for weight loss, 4
and lunch, 96
and pizza, 228
putting on, xv, xviii, 12, 121
and sitting, 70–71, 90
and sleep, 236
and stress, 140
and traveling, 170
and unconventional jobs, 183,
187, 189, 194, 199, 202
problem solving, 8, 13, 26, 48, 56,
76, 133, 144, 148, 156–158, 197
protein
and alcohol, 221
breakfast, 30, 32, 34, 38, 41
lunch, 102–104
and night shift, 199, 201
and overtime, 227–228
portions, 214
post-workout, 44
snacks, 114

Purdue University, 223

Q
quinoa, 110, 216

R
restaurants, 63, 97–98, 104,
108–110, 167, 171, 175, 179,
202, 210, 217–221, 227. *See
also* eating out
Right Management, 94
running, 70–71, 82, 89, 146, 205,
231

S
salad dressing, 103, 107, 128,
200, 206, 219–220, 229
salads, 102–103, 106–107,
109–111, 119, 128–130,
170, 180, 192, 200, 206, 217,
228–229
Salk Institute for Biological
Studies, 159
salmon, 102, 105, 170
salt, sodium, 17, 34, 40, 129, 200,
218, 222
sandwiches, 39–40, 103, 105,
109, 110–111, 121, 129, 163,
170, 189, 192, 219
serotonin, 189
sitting
and commuting, 48–49, 51–
52, 57–58, 63, 184
and exercising, 52–58, 82–87.
See also desk workouts

preventing problems of,
72–80, 87–93, 133–135

and side effects, 69–72,
111–112

and weight gain, xvii, 51, 70

sleep

and health, 49, 143, 157–159,
191, 233–234, 236–237.
See also napping

strategies for, 169, 194–195,
229, 237–240

and technology, 235

and weight, 49, 235–236

and work, 25–26, 190, 192,
195, 197–199, 237

smartphone. *See* phone

smoothies, 41, 44

snacks

BYO, 166–168, 204–205

and commuting, 61–62, 66–67

and coworkers, 7, 20

and events, 120

happy hours, 221–224

healthy choices, 5, 44, 62,
114–115, 189, 199–210,
215, 230, 239

and lunch, 110, 113–115

and long hours, 209, 227

and per diem, 170

portion size, 214

and vending machines, 198

soy milk, 32, 41, 198

spinning, 42, 231

standing desks and risers, 88–90

Stanford University, 76, 135

strategies. *See also* management;
planning

for breakfast, 24, 28–29, 33,
37, 42

for commuting, 54

for dinner, 215–217, 219,
230–231, 233

for lunch, 100–102, 114

for happy hours, 223–224

for stress management, 147,
152, 155–162

for traveling, 165–166,
172–173, 176, 179, 181

for unconventional jobs,
182–183, 192, 194–198,
205–206

for sleeping, 237–240

for work, xvii, 3–6, 8, 13–14,
20–21, 75, 80, 124, 129,
131, 227–228, 241

strawberries, 32, 105, 114, 204

stress

background, 140–143

and commuting, 49–50,
52–53, 58–62, 64, 184

cortisol (stress hormone),
146–147

damage of, 143–145

managing, 26, 137, 147–148,
152–162, 188

and night shift work, 193–194,
193, 195, 198

stressors, 141, 148–151, 183,
211, 230, 234

stroke, 28, 31, 34, 130, 143, 228, 236

substitutions, 14, 37, 40–41, 103, 129, 175, 180, 219–220

sugar
   and alcohol, 223
   and breakfast, 23, 27, 31–32, 34–39, 41, 43
   and commuting, 50–51, 62–63
   and dinner, 218
   and events, 117, 120–122, 124, 130, 132
   foods at work, 2–6, 10–12, 14, 17–18
   and lunch, 105, 114
   and long hours, 227, 229
   and sleep deprivation, 236
   and stress, 146–147
   and traveling, 169
   and unconventional jobs, 194, 196–198

sugar-free options, 5, 14–15, 39–40, 129, 198

superfood, 102, 105, 114

swimming, 176–177

T

takeout, 164, 219

tea, 37, 105, 169, 173, 192–193, 201

teamwork, 116, 121–122, 125, 128, 131, 133, 135, 138–139, 153, 178, 184

technology, 6, 24, 95, 165, 183, 211, 235

telecommuting, 66, 184–190, 207

telomeres, 130

Temple University, 236

texting, 59, 67, 69, 177, 183, 235, 238

theanine, 169

tofu, 41, 199–200, 216

tomatoes, 13, 102–103, 107, 129, 216, 224, 228–229

trans fat, 11, 13, 129

traveling, 163–171, 175, 181

treadmill, 43, 176

treadmill desks, 89–90

tuna, 102–103, 105, 115, 189, 200

TV, 162, 177, 212–213

U

University of Arizona, 99

University of Bath, 26–27

University of California, Irvine, 151

University of California, Berkeley, 235–236

University of Georgia, 157

University of Minnesota, 90

University of Oslo, 138

University of Pennsylvania, 235

University of Rochester Medical Center, 141

University of South Australia, 145

University of Texas Southwest Medical Center, 70

Uppsala University, 35

V

vegan, 14, 110, 175

vegetables

for breakfast, 31, 41
for dinner, 214, 217, 219–220, 228
and events, 130
for lunch, 102–103, 105, 114
as snacks, 114
and traveling, 166, 170, 175, 180
and unconventional jobs, 189, 199–201, 204, 206
vegetarian, 14, 110, 175
vending machines, 2, 8, 26, 100, 114, 192, 198, 200
Virginia Tech Transportation Institute, 67
vitamins, 10, 34–35, 103, 166, 189, 200–201, 220
volunteering, on the job, 160–161

W

walking
  and commuting, 45, 48, 51, 63–65, 139
  and dinner, 232–233
  after eating, 233
  and long hours, 229
  and lunch, 109, 111–112
  and meetings, 7, 75–77
  pedometers, 133–136
  programs, 133–137, 139
  and stress, 157
  traveling, 169, 173, 176
  and unconventional jobs, 190, 195–196

and weight control, 2, 70–71, 73–74, 78–80, 84, 87–90, 93
Washington University in St. Louis, 47, 76
water
  and breakfast, 35
  and commuting, 62
  and happy hours, 222
  and lunch, 105
  and specialty waters, 41, 105
  and traveling, 168, 170, 173
  and unconventional jobs, 197, 201, 203–204
  and workouts, 44
  at the workplace, 77
websites, 9, 39, 60, 65, 132, 138, 165, 167, 190, 219, 232
weight loss competitions, 138–139
weight loss goals, setting, 4–5
weight loss tools, 714
weightlifting, 58, 86, 177
wellness, 42, 46, 48, 90, 115, 134–137, 153, 195
Wheeling Jesuit University, 61
whole grains
  bagels, 13
  breakfast, 34, 40, 44
  dinner, 219, 228
  lunch, 103, 129–130, 189
  sandwich options, 103
  and sleeping, 239
  travel, 169
whole wheat, 13, 34. *See also* whole grains

WiFi, 24, 169, 177
wine, 169, 178, 223
Work Stress Survey, 140
working from home, 67, 182–190
workout. *See* exercise

Y

yoga, 42–43, 137–138, 156, 177,
    233
yogurt
    and breakfast, 38–39
    frozen, 107, 165–166

Greek, 38, 41, 44
and morning workout, 44
in smoothies, 41
as snack, 114–115, 201, 230
while traveling, 165–166
at work, 15, 130, 206